WO
710
WEL

For Elsevier

Commissioning Editor: *Timothy Horne*
Development Editor: *Helen Leng*
Project Manager: *Glenys Norquay*
Designer: *Charles Gray*
Illustration Manager: *Bruce Hogarth*
Illustrator: *Richard Tibbitts, Paul Richardson*

LOCAL AND REGIONAL ANAESTHESIA IN THE EMERGENCY DEPARTMENT

MADE EASY

Mike Wells MBBCh MScMed(Emergency Medicine) Dip PEC(SA) FCEM(SA)
Specialist Emergency Physician
Lecturer and Consultant
Division of Emergency Medicine
Faculty of Health Sciences
University of the Witwatersrand
and
Netcare Union Hospital Emergency Department
Johannesburg
South Africa

Contributor
Lara Goldstein MBBCh FCEM(SA)
Specialist Emergency Physician
Division of Emergency Medicine
Faculty of Health Sciences
University of the Witwatersrand
and
Gauteng Emergency Medical Services
Johannesburg
South Africa

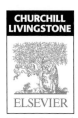

CHURCHILL LIVINGSTONE

ELSEVIER

Edinburgh   London   New York   Oxford   Philadelphia   St Louis   Sydney   Toronto 2010

CHURCHILL
LIVINGSTONE
ELSEVIER

© 2010 Elsevier Ltd All rights reserved.

ISBN 9780702034886
International ISBN 9780702034879

British Library Cataloguing in Publication Data
A catalogue record for this book is available from the British Library

Library of Congress Cataloging in Publication Data
A catalog record for this book is available from the Library of Congress

Notices
Knowledge and best practice in this field are constantly changing. As new research and experience broaden our understanding, changes in research methods, professional practices or medical treatment may become necessary.

Practitioners and researchers must always rely on their own experience and knowledge in evaluating and using any information, methods, compounds, or experiments described herein. In using such information or methods they should be mindful of their own safety and the safety of others, including parties for whom they have a professional responsibility.

With respect to any drug or pharmaceutical products identified, readers are advised to check the most current information provided (i) on procedures featured or (ii) by the manufacturer of each product to be administered, to verify the recommended dose or formula, the method and duration of administration, and contraindications. It is the responsibility of practitioners, relying on their own experience and knowledge of their patients, to make diagnoses, to determine dosages and the best treatment for each individual patient, and to take all appropriate safety precautions.

To the fullest extent of the law, neither the publisher nor the authors, contributors or editors assume any liability for any injury and/or damage to persons or property as a matter of products liability, negligence or otherwise, or from any use or operation of any methods, products, instructions or ideas contained in the material herein.

ELSEVIER your source for books, journals and multimedia in the health sciences
www.elsevierhealth.com

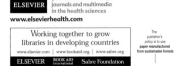

Working together to grow libraries in developing countries
www.elsevier.com | www.bookaid.org | www.sabre.org

ELSEVIER   BOOK AID International   Sabre Foundation

The publisher's policy is to use paper manufactured from sustainable forests

Printed in China

Contents

Contents

Acknowledgements

Any sort of work like this is dependent on many people for its completion. I am grateful to all the people I love for their help, support and forbearance while this project was underway.

In addition to her chapter in the book, I am especially grateful to Dr Lara Goldstein for advice, assistance, proofreading and many hours of discussion. Much obliged indeed!

Images were obtained from the following machines:

- Medison Pico (kindly lent by SSEM Mthembu as arranged by Heidi Richter).
- Siemens Acuson X300 (kindly lent by Siemens South Africa as arranged by Tanya Reynolds).
- Philips HD 11XE (kindly lent by Netcare Union Hospital).

The images of the probe are from a Toshiba Nemio 10 linear 5 to 12 MHz transducer which is the workhorse of the ED, again kindly lent by Netcare Union Hospital.

Figs 4.1, 4.4, 4.7, 8.1, 8.31A–C, 8.56A&B, 9.1, 9.10A–C, 9.22A–C, 9.38A–C adapted from Gray's Atlas of Anatomy. Richard Drake, A. Wayne Vogl, Adam Mitchell, Richard Tibbitts, Paul Richardson. ISBN 13: 9780443067211.

Preface

One of the most common reasons for patients to present to the emergency department (ED) is pain. Therefore one of the key objectives of patient management in the ED is the rapid and effective treatment of pain and alleviation of associated anxiety. Likewise, it is important to minimise patient discomfort (or pain) and apprehension during ED procedures. These are core skills needed especially by emergency physicians but also by other doctors involved in acute patient management. A sound knowledge of the drugs, procedures and techniques, as well as the equipment and staffing prerequisites, is essential.

The key to the successful use of procedural sedation and local anaesthesia (in any of its applications) is patience:

- The slow injection of subcutaneous local anaesthetic over 10 seconds is much less painful than the same volume given over 2 seconds.
- It takes several minutes for the development of complete anaesthesia following local infiltration; sedative and analgesic agents take some time to work to achieve optimum effect.
- The ED is often a hurried and harried environment, but keeping patients waiting *at the right time* (e.g. for the EMLA patch to work) will result in far higher patient (or parent) satisfaction.

This book was designed not so much to teach new ideas or practices, but to remind you of the things that you have already learnt, and to share some practical tips on aspects of patient management that might not be found in textbooks. The exact landmarks for a block are easily forgotten and a quick reference to look them up can be very useful. If you haven't had some training in ultrasound nerve blocks then this book won't teach you how to do them, but it will help you if you haven't done one for a while. Some of the procedures here are very easy, while other procedures are trickier and should be attempted only in the correct teaching environment with adequate supervision. I have made extensive use of pictures to illustrate the landmarks and needle puncture sites, and ultrasound images from two different patients – a muscular male and a slim female. All blocks have been illustrated being performed on the RIGHT side, unless otherwise indicated.

The use of both regional anaesthesia and procedural sedation in the ED are mildly controversial, mostly because of concerns about their safety. There is no doubt, however, that the evidence supports the appropriate use of these techniques. ED physicians are trained to deal with any of the potential side effects or complications that may arise: they are experienced in the management of airway emergencies, ventilation, cardiovascular emergencies, and neurological emergencies. ED physicians generally also have had training in anaesthesia, which should encompass basic nerve-block techniques, including the use of nerve stimulators. They are often familiar with basic emergency ultrasound, which makes the use of ultrasound for nerve blocks a much easier skill to acquire.

Analgesia in the ED has the potential to be an extremely elegant aspect of clinical management … or a downright disaster if it is ignored or performed poorly. It is my challenge to you to expertly manage your patients' pain, in the same way that you would like to be treated if you were that patient.

From the paediatric perspective: never forget that children are important! It is too easy to forget that the management of children requires **more** attention to anxiolysis and appropriate analgesia than it might for adults. It is too easy to 'hold the kid down' or 'wrap him tightly' for venesection, intravenous access, suturing or other noxious procedures. Expediency or lack of time is a poor excuse for what is increasingly becoming regarded (and rightly so) as unethical practice. There is a significant body of evidence to show that inadequate attention to early analgesia following trauma and failure to provide good procedural sedation and analgesia (including local anaesthesia) can have long-term psychological and physiological effects in children. It is important to acquire the skill to administer appropriate drugs to infants and children for topical and local anaesthesia and procedural sedation and/or analgesia. It might take a bit more knowledge, a bit longer, but it is possible to avoid much of the iatrogenic screaming emanating from the ED!

CHAPTER 1

Local anaesthesia

The administration of local anaesthetics is indicated whenever their use will ease pain from trauma, or decrease the discomfort of a painful procedure. Local anaesthesia is thus useful in many clinical situations to increase patient comfort and facilitate cooperation during painful procedures. The successful use of local anaesthesia can be maximised by an understanding of the pharmacokinetics of local anaesthetic agents, the indications for their use, appropriate methods of administration and techniques to minimise the pain of administration.

Pharmacology

Local anaesthetics reversibly block nerve impulse conduction by blocking open, voltage-gated sodium channels (and possibly also interfering with calcium channels), thereby inhibiting the action potential; they have additional anti-inflammatory effects mediated through interaction with G-protein receptors.

The onset of action depends on the individual agent and the dose delivered to the nerve. The more lipid soluble (lipophilic/hydrophobic) an agent is, the greater its potency and duration of action. Similarly, the smaller the local anaesthetic molecule is, the faster its dissociation from the receptor and the shorter its duration of action. All local anaesthetics, with the single exception of cocaine, are vasodilators, which increases the clearance of the agent; the addition of adrenaline (epinephrine) in a ratio of 1 : 80 000 to 1 : 400 000 causes optimum vasoconstriction for bleeding control and prolongation of action. The addition of adrenaline to long-acting agents does less to prolong their action

Table 1.1 Local anaesthetics readily available in clinical practice

Agent	Lipid solubility	Duration of action (min)	Time of onset (min)	Maximum dose (mg/kg)	Maximum dose with adrenaline (mg/kg)
Amides					
Bupivacaine	High	200+	10–15	3	3.5–5
Lidocaine	Medium	30–60	5	4.5	7
Mepivacaine	Low	45–90	3	4	
Ropivacaine	Medium	200+	5–15	3	
Esters					
Procaine	Low	40	15–20	7	
Tetracaine	High	200	15	1.5	

than in short-acting agents. The use of adrenaline is traditionally avoided in areas of limited vascular supply (fingers, toes, penis, nose and ears) although there is no evidence to prove that this is in fact harmful. If excessive vasoconstriction occurs, the pH of the interstitial fluid drops, which will result in a decreased activity of the local anaesthetic. It is important, therefore, not to use vasoconstrictors in excessive concentrations (1 : 80 000 or less is most appropriate).

Systemic absorption of the agent depends principally on the vascularity of the injection site. The rate of absorption and the risk of toxicity increase as shown below:

Subcutaneous injection → peripheral nerve blocks →
    brachial plexus blocks → intercostal blocks →
    upper airway administration → intravenous injection.

There are many local anaesthetics readily available in clinical practice (Table 1.1). The most widely used agents include lidocaine and bupivacaine. Local anaesthetics are most commonly used during wound repair and for minor procedures (drainage of abscesses etc.). Techniques for their administration in the ED include topical application, local infiltration, field block, and peripheral nerve block. Lidocaine, the most commonly used local anaesthetic, is inexpensive and is available in a variety of concentrations (1% and 2%) and volumes (20-mL vials, 5-mL ampoules, and 1.8-mL dental cartridges). Some formulations are appropriate for subcutaneous administration only. Only the IV preparation should be used for intravenous regional anaesthesia and haematoma blocks. The combination of 1% or 2% lidocaine with adrenaline in a ratio of 1 : 80 000 (found in dental cartridges or premixed vials) produces optimal skin vasoconstriction and adequate duration of effect for most procedures. If premixed solutions are not available, the addition of 0.1 mL of adrenaline 1 : 1000 to 10 mL of lidocaine will create a 1 : 100 000 solution. Bupivacaine has a much longer duration of action than lidocaine and therefore may be more appropriate for very complex wounds requiring long repair times or when prolonged post-procedure analgesia is required. In settings where wound care may be interrupted (in a busy ED), the use of bupivacaine may avoid the need for further administration of local anaesthesia to complete a wound repair. For these reasons, many ED physicians choose bupivacaine or ropivacaine over lidocaine. A mixture of the two agents is often used because of the rapid onset of lidocaine and the longer duration of bupivacaine and to increase the volume of injected agent for regional anaesthesia. Studies have suggested that bupivacaine is underused in the ED, mostly because it is unfamiliar or because doctors have misconceptions about its onset of action or safety. It is an excellent local anaesthetic for the ED!

Adverse events

Fortunately, true hypersensitivity reactions to local anaesthetics are rare and most commonly involve an ester agent (e.g. procaine, cocaine, tetracaine, benzocaine). Allergic reactions are very seldom caused by amide anaesthetic agents (e.g. lidocaine, bupivacaine, mepivacaine, ropivacaine). There is no cross-reactivity between the amide and ester agents whatsoever. An easy 'rule of thumb' method to distinguish between amide and ester agents is from the spelling convention of the generic name. Any local anaesthetic in which the letter 'i' appears in the prefix of the name is an amide agent (e.g. lidocaine). The ester agents do not contain an 'i' in the prefix (e.g. cocaine, benzocaine, procaine). If a patient is allergic to a particular agent from one class, an agent from the other class can safely be substituted.

Toxic adverse events are dose related; therefore, the maximum dose for any agent should not be exceeded (Table 1.1). Adverse reactions involve the central nervous system (CNS) and, to a lesser degree, the cardiovascular system (CVS).

Use smaller doses in debilitated patients, very young or very old patients, patients who are acutely ill, and those with cardiovascular disease or liver disease. Adrenaline, as an additive, should be avoided in hypertensive patients and those with cardiovascular or ischaemic heart disease.

Decreasing the pain of local anaesthesia

It is important, especially in children, to make the procedure of administering local anaesthesia as atraumatic (physically and psychologically) as possible. The pain of injecting the local anaesthetic is increased by the patient's anxiety and apprehension and this needs to be addressed as carefully as the physical pain itself. The discomfort from the needlestick and from chemical irritation of the agent may be decreased somewhat by the following techniques:

- A thorough discussion of the procedure with patient and parents to decrease anxiety and apprehension.
- Distraction with toys, music, TV, virtual reality devices.
- Sucrose – a sweet can make a big difference!
- Allow an infant to feed with a bottle or on the breast while administering the local anaesthetic, if possible.
- Pressure or rubbing the skin near the injection site can decrease the pain sensation.
- Commercially available 'acupuncture' devices (e.g. the Bionix Shot Blocker) may decrease the perception of pain from a needlestick.
- Dripping local anaesthetic into the wound or the use of topical anaesthetics before injection and the application of lidocaine or tetracaine to mucosal surfaces will induce topical anaesthesia.
- Slow injection of the local anaesthetic agent – a slow injection over 10 seconds is **much** less painful than a fast injection over 2 seconds.
- Superficial injections into the dermis are more painful than injections into the dermal–subcutaneous tissue junction.
- Cold local anaesthetic causes more pain on injection than body temperature solution.
- Increasing the pH of the lidocaine by adding sodium bicarbonate in a 1 : 10 ratio (1 mL $NaHCO_3$ to 10 mL lidocaine 1%) will decrease the pain of injection and also increase the duration of action (increased lipid solubility, decreased vasodilatation and washout).

- Use a long needle (spinal needles work very well) to make as few punctures as possible, and a small gauge to minimise injection pain. Also use the smallest syringe that is appropriate for the volume to be injected – this gives the greatest control over the rate of injection.
- Use peripheral nerve blocks where possible – it is less painful than local infiltration, e.g. a mental block for a lower lip laceration.
- Wait long enough for the infiltration or nerve block anaesthesia to take effect. This may be 5 to 10 minutes for local infiltration and 20 to 30 minutes for nerve blocks. Never begin a procedure immediately after injecting local anaesthetic.

Before injecting the local anaesthetic, make sure of the following:

- The patient must be comfortable and at ease.
- All equipment needed for the local infiltration must be available nearby.
- Appropriate monitoring equipment (if required) should be available.
- Lighting and positioning of the patient must be adequate.
- Resuscitation medications and equipment must be easily accessible.
- Sterile procedures should be followed as much as possible.

For the safety of the healthcare provider, make sure of the following:

- Wear approved eye protection and gloves at all times.
- Practise a safe needle-handling technique.
- Select patients appropriately – intoxicated or confused patients may move unexpectedly, which can increase the risk of needlestick injuries.
- Get informed consent (verbal or written as appropriate) for every procedure.
- Keep good written records of the procedure.

Basic infiltration techniques

Local anaesthesia may be obtained by injecting a local anaesthetic agent directly into the wound or by infiltrating as a field block. Intra-dermal injection has the advantages of a rapid onset of action after injection and an increased duration of anaesthesia compared with that of deeper anaesthetic placement. However, intradermal injection significantly distorts the tissues, and it is more painful than sub-cutaneous injection. For most purposes, local anaesthetic injected at the dermal–subcutaneous junction is ideal: the injection is not too painful and the anaesthetic results are excellent. As a rule, subcutaneous infiltration should not begin until it has been confirmed that the needle has not penetrated a vessel (pull back on the plunger of the syringe to ensure that blood is not aspirated). This technique is not reliable when a 30G needle is used (it is too small for blood to be aspirated).

Direct wound infiltration

Injection through the wound itself into the surrounding skin edges is less painful than injecting through the skin, especially if local anaes-thetic is dripped into the wound beforehand, or if topical anaesthesia is used. Although this theoretically has the risk of transporting bacteria from the wound into the surrounding tissue, this has not been proven to result in a higher complication rate. It would seem appropriate, however, that this should not be performed on a heavily contaminated wound.

Parallel field block

This is more appropriate for complex wounds, contaminated wounds, wounds that require debridement or simple flaps. The needle is inserted at one end of the wound and advanced to the other end of the wound, parallel to it. After aspiration to ensure the needle has not penetrated a vessel, local anaesthetic is injected slowly as the needle is slowly withdrawn. Injection may be in the dermis (superficial anaes-thesia, painful technique) or more commonly at the junction of the dermis and subcutaneous tissue: this takes a bit longer to achieve anaesthesia (5 to 10 minutes), but is less painful. This procedure should be repeated until there are parallel tracks on both sides of the wound.

Circular field block

If the wound is irregular or complex, local anaesthetic can be infiltrated in a circular pattern at some distance from the wound edge, in the same method as described above. This technique is extremely useful for procedures on the ear. A circumference of subcutaneous local anaes-thetic is infiltrated inferior, superior, anterior and posterior to the pinna, which results in complete anaesthesia of the ear.

Special local anaesthetic applications

Local anaesthesia for line placement

The placement of central venous catheters and arterial cannulas can be made less unpleasant with the correct use of local anaesthesia.

Central line technique

- Consider procedural sedation as an adjunct to this procedure.
- Identify the target point for needle insertion and raise a subcutaneous weal of local anaesthetic.
- Infiltrate subcutaneous local anaesthetic at the expected sites of anchor sutures.
- Insert the needle along the tract to be followed to access the central vein and inject local anaesthetic while withdrawing the needle. Aspirate frequently to exclude accidental intravascular injection.

Arterial line technique

- Consider procedural sedation as an adjunct to this procedure.
- In children especially, use an EMLA patch over the site of anticipated cannulation and leave on for at least 60 minutes.
- Identify and mark the pulsation of the artery to be cannulated.
- Raise a small weal of local anaesthetic subcutaneously at the site at which the cannula is to be inserted.
- Inject small (0.5 mL) volumes of local anaesthetic on each side of the artery proximal to the site of puncture; larger volumes will distort the anatomy and make palpation difficult.

Local anaesthesia for intercostal drain insertion

In the ED, chest drain insertion may be emergent (pneumothorax, haemothorax) or semi-emergent (pleural effusion, empyema or spontaneous pneumothorax). While the type of procedural sedation used may vary, the administration of the local anaesthetic remains much the same.

Technique

- Consider procedural sedation with this procedure, particularly if the thoracostomy is not an emergency procedure.
- Identify the site for intercostal drain insertion (normally the 5th intercostal space just anterior to the midaxillary line).

- Raise a subcutaneous weal of local anaesthetic.
- Advance the needle through the tissue layers while injecting (after aspirating to exclude intravascular needle placement). Aim to penetrate the pleura on the superior aspect of the 6th rib, to avoid the neurovascular bundle which runs on the inferior aspect of the rib above.
- Repeat this in a fan shape, aiming to pierce the pleura in several spots around the intended course of dissection. Use a full 20 mL of 1% lidocaine for this infiltration.
- Once the drain has been placed, consider an intrapleural block.
- As an alternative, intercostal nerve blocks of the 4th, 5th and 6th ribs may be performed.

Local anaesthesia for lumbar puncture

Lumbar punctures can be rendered virtually painless by the correct administration of local anaesthetic. The recurrent spinal nerves exit the neural foramina and travel posteriorly to supply sensation to the posterior spinal structures. These nerves can easily be blocked. Lumbar puncture should always be performed with local anaesthesia and with procedural sedation (light sedation) if required, especially in children.

Technique

- Apply a topical anaesthetic agent (e.g. EMLA cream or patch) to the area to be injected (if necessary). Allow sufficient time for this to become effective before proceeding.
- Position the patient correctly to identify the landmarks.
- Clean the target area with an antiseptic solution and position sterile drapes as needed.
- Raise a subcutaneous weal of local anaesthetic over the interspace to be used. Administer another weal superficial to a second interspace above or below the one to be used.
- Introduce the needle and advance it to the interspinous ligament and inject 0.5 to 1 mL of local anaesthetic; advance the needle slightly deeper and inject a further 0.5 mL of anaesthetic.
- Withdraw the needle to the subcutaneous tissue and redirect it to either side of the spinous process; inject 3 to 4 mL of local anaesthetic on each side to block the recurrent spinal nerves.

CHAPTER 2

Local anaesthetic toxidromes and complications

Local complications

Local complications are usually a result of the injection technique. Immediate complications include pain, bruising, haematoma formation, local skin reactions (dermatitis) and nerve injury. Delayed complications include infection, complicated haematomas and neurapraxias.

- Tissue irritation caused by local anaesthetics is generally related to the acidity of the infiltrated solution and there are ways to minimise this discomfort, which will be discussed later.
- Ecchymoses or haematomas are a result of the perforation of cutaneous or subcutaneous blood vessels. This may be more severe in patients with a bleeding disorder (inherent or acquired as a result of medications: aspirin, clopidogrel or other anticoagulants). If bruising occurs, the patient can simply be reassured. A significant haematoma may require drainage and a pressure dressing, but this is an extremely rare complication.
- EMLA and other topical anaesthetics can cause itching, burning, pain, pallor, erythema, oedema, and purpura. Irritant dermatitis, allergic contact dermatitis, and contact urticaria can also occur.

- Nerve injury may occur during the infiltration of a local anaesthetic. This may occur from nerve laceration by the needle or nerve contusion by intraneural injection. This complication occurs more commonly during the performance of regional blocks than local infiltration. Clinical indications of potential nerve injury include paraesthesias, 'electric shock' sensations and excessive pain during needle insertion, advancement or injection. Withdraw the needle and reposition it should this happen. The majority of neurapraxias resolve over a period of a few days or weeks.
- Nerve injury might also result from an excessively high concentration of local anaesthetic. For this reason, lower concentrations are preferred (bupivacaine 0.5% or lower, ropivacaine 0.5% or lower, lidocaine 2% or lower).
- Acute myotoxicity may be associated with local anaesthetics, but has only been reported following continuous peripheral nerve blocks.
- Infection is a potential complication of any injection. It occurs most commonly as a complication of haematoma formation. Maintain sterile conditions as much as possible, and ensure appropriate treatment of haematomas. Many studies have shown that these procedures are not truly sterile, but need to be as clean as possible. Extra care must be taken with patients who are immunocompromised.

Systemic complications

Systemic complications include hypersensitivity reactions, anaphylaxis and toxicity of the local anaesthetic agent.

Allergic reactions, in all forms, are idiosyncratic and can occur at any dose. They are more common with the ester local anaesthetics, but can occur with any medication. Allergic reactions can be in response to the local anaesthetic agent or to the preservative agent (e.g. methyl hydroxybenzoate). Anaphylactic reactions should be treated with intramuscular adrenaline (epinephrine) (0.5 mg in the anterolateral thigh for adults), intravenous fluids, intravenous steroids (e.g. hydro-cortisone 4 mg/kg) and possibly intravenous antihistamines (e.g. pro-methazine 0.5 mg/kg). Resuscitation equipment should always be available in an environment where local or regional anaesthesia is practised.

Methaemoglobinaemia may be caused by any local anaesthetic agent, but prilocaine is the most common culprit, especially in children.

Methaemoglobinaemia can produce clinically significant hypoxaemia and can interfere with pulse oximetry, producing an exaggeratedly low saturation figure (around 85%). Treatment is with intravenous methylene blue 1 mg/kg.

Systemic adverse effects usually occur when blood concentrations of local anaesthetic increase to toxic levels. These effects are most often encountered after inadvertent intravenous injection, systemic release of local anaesthetic after intravenous regional anaesthesia, or administration of an excessive dose of a local anaesthetic or topical agent (especially on broken skin or mucous membranes). Patients in the ED are particularly at risk since the trauma patient may get local anaesthetic for the placement of an intercostal drain, for the central venous catheter, for wound repair, topical anaesthesia of the upper airway, an intrapleural block and so on.

Patients with decreased pseudocholinesterase activity are more susceptible to toxicity from ester anaesthetics and patients who are taking medications that inhibit the cytochrome P450 system (e.g. propofol, amiodarone, ciprofloxacin, macrolides, tricyclic antidepressants, selective serotonin reuptake inhibitors, cimetidine, imidazole antifungals, antiepileptic medications, benzodiazepines, beta blockers, calcium channel blockers, statins, immunosuppressants, and antiviral agents) are more susceptible to toxicity from amide anaesthetics.

The systemic toxicity of local anaesthetic agents affects the central nervous system (CNS) and the cardiovascular system. CNS lidocaine toxicity is biphasic and as the serum levels of lidocaine increases, the effects on the CNS become more severe. The first phase of side effects occurs as a result of CNS excitation and can include irritability and seizures. The second phase causes CNS depression. The seizures stop (and not because the patient is getting better) and coma and respiratory depression or arrest may develop. This biphasic effect occurs because local anaesthetics first block inhibitory CNS pathways (resulting in stimulation) and then eventually block both inhibitory and excitatory pathways (resulting in overall CNS inhibition).

- At mildly toxic lidocaine levels, patients may experience tinnitus, light-headedness, perioral numbness, diplopia, a metallic taste in the mouth, nausea and/or vomiting, or they may become loquacious.
- As serum levels increase, nystagmus, dysarthria, localised muscle twitching, or fine tremors may be noticed. Hallucinations may occur.

- Progressive toxicity may cause focal seizure activity followed by generalised tonic–clonic seizures.
- Respiratory depression and coma follow with extremely high levels.

Resuscitation of these patients should follow a standard Advanced Life Support algorithm (the ABCD approach) with an emphasis on avoiding hypoxia, hypercapnia and acidaemia as this increases the toxicity of local anaesthetics. Seizures should be managed with intravenous benzodiazepines (e.g. lorazepam or diazepam). Significant persistent neurological abnormalities have not been documented following seizures induced by local anaesthetic toxicity.

Many of the adverse effects affecting the cardiovascular system that occur with the administration of local anaesthetics may be as a result of the addition of adrenaline rather than direct effects of the anaesthetic itself (such as tachycardia and hypertension). However, high blood levels of local anaesthetics directly reduce cardiac contractility and cause vasodilatation, which can result in hypotension. Atrioventricular blocks, bradycardia, and ventricular arrhythmias can occur; but these are more common in patients with underlying conduction abnormalities. The management of hypotension should be symptomatic with intravenous fluids (e.g. warm Ringer's lactate or Balsol) and vasopressors used as needed (ephedrine for transient hypotension and adrenaline for sustained hypotension). Hypertension should be treated with intravenous benzodiazepines, and not any other medications. Ventricular tachycardia should be treated with amiodarone. Most other arrhythmias require only symptomatic treatment.

Cardiac arrest following local anaesthetic toxicity that is refractive to conventional resuscitation techniques may respond to treatment with a lipid emulsion – there are case reports of success with this protocol: a 1.5 mL/kg bolus of a 20% solution over 1 minute, followed by an infusion at a rate of 0.25 mL/kg/min. The bolus may be repeated twice every 3 to 5 minutes or until the return of spontaneous circulation. The infusion should be continued until haemodynamic stability is achieved and the rate increased to 0.5 mL/kg/min if the blood pressure drops. A total dose of 8 mL/kg should not be exceeded. If lipid emulsion is not available, an induction dose of propofol (which is buffered in a 13% lipid emulsion) followed by an infusion may be considered instead.

CHAPTER 3

Topical anaesthesia

Topical anaesthesia is an extremely useful adjunct to clinical practice in the ED and is underutilised, often because it is forgotten. It is used for local anaesthesia or analgesia on intact skin, mucous membranes and the eye through the application of local anaesthetic agents to the external epithelial surface. Topical agents may be used to decrease the pain and discomfort of medical procedures and for various skin and mucous membrane conditions, including pruritus and pain due to minor trauma, burns or inflammatory conditions affecting the skin (e.g. varicella, sunburn, contact dermatitis, insect bites).

Do not forget to ask patients about local anaesthetic allergies, as ester-linked agents (which more commonly provoke reactions) are often used for topical anaesthesia.

Cryoanaesthesia

Thermal anaesthesia (cryoanaesthesia) may be used for short-acting superficial anaesthesia for procedures such as venipuncture, intravenous cannula placement, and superficial abscess incision and drainage. Ice, refrigerant sprays and liquid nitrogen have been used for this purpose. This technique does not produce very good anaesthesia.

Technique

- Ice must be applied to the skin for at least 30 to 60 seconds before the procedure. Be careful to avoid frostbite.
- Ethyl chloride may be sprayed onto the skin for 5 to 10 seconds from a distance of about 150 to 200 mm. After a frost is produced on the skin, a 10- to 12-second period of anaesthesia occurs before the skin temperature and sensation return to normal. As a result of this limited time frame, an assistant often has to spray the area while the procedure is performed. Be careful to avoid freezing areas of normal skin by overuse of this method.

Dermal topical local anaesthesia

Topical anaesthesia to the skin is a very useful but underused form of local anaesthesia in the ED. If used correctly, it can dramatically decrease the pain and anxiety associated with injections and other minor procedures.

EMLA (eutectic mixture of local anaesthetics) cream is a combination of lidocaine and prilocaine which has good skin penetration and produces excellent anaesthesia of the skin. Anaesthesia to a depth of 3 mm is obtained after 60 minutes of application under an occlusive dressing, while after 120 minutes the depth of anaesthesia may reach a maximum of 5 mm. The onset of action may be more rapid in highly vascular areas (such as the face), and in damaged or inflamed skin. The maximum dose should never be exceeded. EMLA produces a biphasic vascular effect – vasoconstriction followed after 30 minutes of application by vasodilatation.

EMLA cream may be used to decrease the discomfort of vascular access, injections, lumbar puncture or superficial procedures. In children, while EMLA certainly has a role in minor procedures, it must be remembered that cooperation has as much to do with apprehension as it does with actual pain, so additional agents or methods may be needed to address this. EMLA cream may be applied under an occlusive dressing or as a pre-prepared product. EMLA should be used for small applications only, because of the toxicity of prilocaine, especially in children (principally methaemoglobinaemia). The maximum dose should not be exceeded (Table 3.1).

Recent studies have suggested that EMLA is safe even in neonates. At this stage, however, this would be an off-label application.

Table 3.1   Recommended dosages of EMLA for children

Age and body weight	Maximum dose (g)	Maximum area (cm²)	Maximum no. of patches
1 to 3 months or <5 kg	1	10	1
4 to 12 months and >5 kg	2	20	2
1 to 6 years and >10 kg	10	100	10
7 to 12 years and >20 kg	20	200	20

Technique

- Prepare the skin prior to application by cleaning with an alcohol swab to degrease the skin.
- Penetration of the topical anaesthetic agent can be increased in intact skin by partially removing the stratum corneum by tape-stripping: apply an adhesive tape to the skin and rip it off in a 'waxing' manoeuvre. Do not traumatise children by causing pain with this procedure.
- Apply EMLA directly to skin with coverage of 1.5 g/10 cm² in adults and 1 g/10 cm² in children and cover with an occlusive dressing, or use a commercially prepared self-adhesive disc.
- Wait sufficient time to achieve the desired depth of anaesthesia (60 minutes = 3 mm, 90 minutes = 4 mm, 120 minutes = 5 mm). If large amounts of cream are still on the skin surface, insufficient time has been allowed for its absorption. A shorter waiting time is required when EMLA is applied on irritated or broken skin.

TAC (tetracaine 0.5%, adrenaline [epinephrine] 0.05% and cocaine 5–12%) has been used as an anaesthetic for repair of facial and scalp lacerations in children, but today sufficient concern exists about toxic potential that it should not be used.

Other options include LAT (lidocaine 4%, adrenaline 0.1% and tetracaine 0.5%) which is prepared as a premixed gel. Where it is not available, a similar mixture can be improvised:

Ophthalmic tetracaine 1% 0.9 mL
Lidocaine 2% 0.9 mL
Adrenaline 1 : 1000 0.2 mL.

Because of the vasoconstrictor effects it should not be used on the fingers, penis, nose or ears. Topical anaesthesia should be used with care on broken skin or mucous membranes and the patient carefully monitored for adverse reactions.

The ophthalmological preparation of tetracaine 1% can be used for topical anaesthesia on its own, especially on mucous membranes (e.g. in the mouth prior to injection for dental anaesthesia).

Lidocaine 2% gel may provide good topical anaesthesia to open wounds and damaged skin ('roasties') but is of little value on intact skin. Do not exceed the maximum permitted dose of 10 mL on broken skin, and 15 mL on mucosa at any one time!

Other formulations and methods

Other preparations include topical liposomal lidocaine formulations and heat-enhanced delivery systems (usually lidocaine and tetracaine preparations). Other needle-free devices for administering local anaesthetic have shown promise and new products will continue to appear. Emergency physicians should be aware of new developments in order to make their patient's visit as minimally unpleasant as possible.

Ophthalmological applications

The ophthalmic division of the trigeminal nerve supplies the cornea, conjunctiva and sclera, via a terminal network of nerves that lies in proximity to the external surface of the eye. Local anaesthesia is therefore very effective in the eye (cataract surgery can be performed with topical anaesthesia alone).

Topical anaesthesia of the eye is useful in the ED:

- To facilitate tonometry.
- For removal of foreign bodies in the cornea and/or conjunctiva.
- For superficial curettage of the cornea (removal of burn rings or 'rust' rings).
- To allow thorough eye lavage to remove chemical or mechanical foreign materials.
- In conjunction with other topical agents for procedures on the eyelids or eyelid margins.
- As a single application in photokeratitis ('arc eyes' or snow blindness) to reduce blepharospasm and allow comprehensive examination of the eye and administration of other agents.

Ester-linked local anaesthetics (such as tetracaine and oxybuprocaine) have traditionally been used in the eye because of their rapid absorption and onset of action within 5 to 10 seconds, and duration of action of 10 to 20 minutes. Amides such as lidocaine and bupivacaine have become more popular because of their longer duration of action, despite their slower absorption. Buffered solutions of lidocaine or bupivacaine have a significantly longer duration of anaesthesia than ester agents, with an onset of action within 1 minute of instillation, and duration of action of 45–60 minutes for lidocaine, and 60–180 minutes for bupivacaine. There is no general consensus on which topical local anaesthetic eye drop provides the best analgesia, but studies have shown that proxymetacaine causes the least discomfort on administration. Tetracaine, oxybuprocaine, proxymetacaine, lidocaine and bupivacaine have all been used successfully in a variety of different concentrations. Availability may determine the choice of agent, but it is essential that the preparation is preservative-free. Increasing the preparation pH (buffering 1 mL of local anaesthetic with 0.1 mL of sodium bicarbonate [1 : 10]) may alter the duration of action but is probably of little clinical benefit in general. Topical non-steroidal anti-inflammatory drugs, such as ketorolac or diclofenac, may be co-administered with local anaesthetics and prescribed for follow-on outpatient treatment for traumatic eye discomfort. Topical steroids should in general only be used in consultation with an ophthalmologist.

Topical local anaesthetic drops should *never* be prescribed for patients' own use for three main reasons:

- When used excessively, topical anaesthetics can cause severe and irreversible damage to corneal tissues, with corneal 'melting'.
- Local anaesthesia increases the likelihood of unnoticed trauma to the cornea from rubbing or foreign bodies – for this reason, every patient discharged from the ED should wear an eye patch on the eye/s that have been anaesthetised, until normal sensation in the eye returns;
- Other causes of pain in the eye (ocular or extraocular) may be masked by the use of topical anaesthesia.

Technique

- Instil drops directly into the affected eye; do not drop the local anaesthetic directly onto the cornea but rather into the inferior fornix of the conjunctiva.
- Follow up with additional drops every few minutes if deeper or prolonged anaesthesia is needed (especially with amide agents). More than five drops will seldom be needed in each eye.

Mucosal topical anaesthetic applications

Topical anaesthesia is very effective when applied to the mucous membranes of the ears, nose, throat, oral cavity, upper airway and genital mucosa because of its rapid absorption. For the same reason, the toxic potential of the local anaesthetic agent is high and the maximum dose should be strictly observed. Administration of topical anaesthetics should be performed with accuracy to ensure that a predetermined amount of drug is administered to allow for the intended effect while minimising the risk of toxicity.

Techniques

- *Intraoral injections and procedures*: in the oral cavity, topical anaesthesia is rapidly obtained by holding a pledget (or cotton bud) soaked in lidocaine 2% or tetracaine 1% against the area to be anaesthetised for 30 seconds.
- *Nasal procedures and packing*: topical anaesthesia of the nose for cauterisation, packing or foreign body removal is best obtained with a 4% solution of cocaine (or lidocaine in higher concentrations). Apply the solution to a pledget and hold it in place against the mucosa for several minutes. Excellent local anaesthesia with vasoconstriction will last for 30 to 60 minutes. Do not exceed the maximum dose of 3 mg/kg (±4 mL of the 4% solution in adults). Lidocaine spray can also be applied to the nasal mucosa for topical anaesthesia; it has the disadvantage of producing vasodilatation which may increase the risk of bleeding from the mucosa.
- *Passage of nasogastric tubes; awake endotracheal intubation, or to blunt the autonomic response to intubation in high-risk patients; endoscopy and bronchoscopy*: topical lidocaine spray is available as a metered dose spray (10 mg/0.1 mL spray) for application in the nose, mouth and throat. The maximum dose to be administered as a topical agent is 200 mg (20 sprays), because of the potential for rapid systemic absorption and toxicity. Benzocaine sprays have largely been replaced by lidocaine sprays because of the concern of methaemoglobinaemia with the use of benzocaine. Inhalations of nebulised lidocaine or bupivacaine are often used, but there is little published evidence to support this practice, and there are concerns about excessive and rapid systemic absorption. It is also probably not as effective as other topical applications. Pledgets

soaked in local anaesthetic which are passed into the posterior nasal space above and below the inferior turbinate can be left in place for several minutes. This will result in anaesthesia to the entire nasal passage and proximal pharynx. Bilateral placement increases the success of the anaesthesia.

- *Procedures involving the external ear canal*: topical anaesthesia of the ear canal can be achieved with ear drops containing benzocaine or procaine (adhere to maximum doses); administer four to five drops into the ear canal and allow several minutes for anaesthesia to develop. EMLA cream has been used in the external ear canal with good effect, but the manufacturer warns that it should not be used if it can migrate into the middle ear (perforation of the tympanic membrane) as it has ototoxic effects in animal models.

- *Placement of urethral catheters*: lidocaine gel 2% provides rapid, excellent anaesthesia to the mucosa of the genital tract for the insertion of urethral catheters. It should *always* be used, especially in males. Do not exceed the maximum dose of 15 mL for mucosal application in adults.

CHAPTER 4

Basic dental and oral local anaesthesia

Dental pain is best managed by a dentist because a dentist knows about teeth and most doctors do not. They can also provide definitive care in an appropriate setting with the correct instruments. Dentists are often not available, however, so patients with toothache or dental injuries often present to the ED for pain relief. Although conventional analgesics are effective, performing a nerve block with a long-acting local anaesthetic will make the patient your friend for life. Dental blocks are also a good choice for pregnant women because local anaesthetics and adrenaline (epinephrine) are not teratogenic and can be administered safely without systemic side effects, if used correctly.

The maxillary dentition receives innervation from the maxillary branch of the trigeminal nerve (anterior, middle and posterior superior alveolar nerves, palatine nerves), and the mandibular dentition from the mandibular division of the trigeminal nerve (inferior alveolar nerve, accessory innervation).

Local anaesthesia for the maxillary dentition

Supraperiosteal or infiltration local anaesthesia

The maxillary teeth are innervated via a network of nerves originating from the maxillary nerve and the infraorbital nerve (Fig. 4.1). These nerves run in the cancellous bone of the maxilla, superior to the roots of the maxillary teeth. The lateral cortical plate of the maxillary alveolus is usually sufficiently thin and porous to allow for effective infiltration (supraperiosteal) local anaesthesia. This technique is not recommended for more than two adjacent teeth or when local infection or inflammation is present. To accomplish this, local anaesthetic is infiltrated along the buccal-gingival fold adjacent to the area to be blocked (e.g. adjacent to the first molar if that tooth is painful from infection or injury).

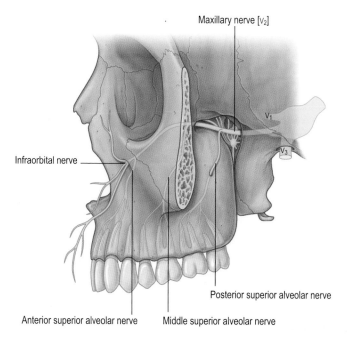

Fig. 4.1 The maxillary nerve and its terminal branches: maxillary nerve, posterior superior alveolar nerve, infraorbital nerve, anterior superior alveolar nerves, middle superior alveolar nerves.

Technique

- Identify the target area for needle insertion – the apex of the buccal-gingival fold adjacent to the target tooth or teeth.
- Dry the mucosa of the target area and apply topical anaesthesia with a cotton bud. Use lidocaine 4% gel or any other topical anaesthetic (improvising with an ester such as tetracaine, which can usually be found amongst the ophthalmic medications, works extremely well).
- Wait 30 seconds for the topical anaesthesia to take effect. To reduce the pain of injection, lift the lip, pull it taut and shake it as the needle is inserted.
- Align the syringe parallel to the long axis of the tooth. With the bevel facing the bone, insert the needle into the target area and advance the needle until the bevel is at or beyond the apex of the tooth (usually just a few millimetres) (Fig. 4.2). There should be no resistance or patient discomfort during this procedure.
- If two teeth need to be blocked, insert the needle of the syringe parallel to the maxillary buccal mucogingival line (where the cheek mucosa reflects onto the gum) opposite the teeth to be anaesthetised (Fig. 4.3).
- Aspirate, and if there is no flashback of blood, inject about 2 to 4 mL of local anaesthetic slowly over 30 to 60 seconds, and continue whilst slowly withdrawing the needle.
- The patient should experience numbness within 2 to 5 minutes of injection. Failure to reach the apex of the tooth when injecting anaesthetic results in varying degrees of soft-tissue numbness without anaesthesia of the tooth itself. If the first attempt at

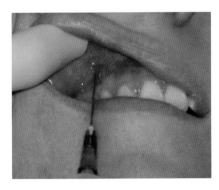

Fig. 4.2 Supraperiosteal infiltration for a single maxillary tooth. The needle is inserted at the apex of the buccal-gingival fold and advanced several millimetres before injecting local anaesthetic.

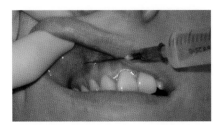

Fig. 4.3 Supraperiosteal infiltration for two or three maxillary teeth. The needle is inserted at the apex of the buccal-gingival fold and advanced posteriorly across the teeth to be blocked. After aspirating, local anaesthetic is injected as the needle is slowly withdrawn.

infiltration fails to provide adequate pain relief, the procedure can safely be repeated several times provided that the total amount of local anaesthetic injected is within the recommended limits.

- Lidocaine provides about 1 hour of dental analgesia and 3 to 5 hours of soft-tissue analgesia. For temporary relief of pain in the ED, the preferred agent is 0.5% bupivacaine or 0.5% ropivacaine with 1 : 200 000 adrenaline. This provides 1 to 3 hours of dental analgesia and 4 to 9 hours of soft-tissue analgesia. The duration of analgesia is less with supraperiosteal infiltration than with regional nerve blocks. The onset of analgesia is within 3 to 10 minutes, depending on which agent is used.

Tips for the non-dentist

- The orientation of the bevel is important in order to decrease the pain of injection and to control the deflection of the needle. When infiltrating, it is better to orientate the bevel towards the bone to avoid scraping the periosteum (Fig. 4.4). It is also important to remember, especially with nerve blocks, that the tip of the needle is deflected away from the side of the bevel as it passes through the tissues. This may amount to as much as 4 mm of deflection in a 30G needle inserted 25 mm into the tissues.
- One cartridge of local anaesthetic (1.8 to 2 mL) is sufficient in dental anaesthesia to provide anaesthesia to most areas. Larger volumes injected over a larger area increase the likelihood of successful anaesthesia, however, especially for the non-expert. The disadvantage of this is the potential for toxic effects of the local anaesthetic and maximum doses should be carefully calculated and observed.
- If local infiltration is ineffective for the maxillary tooth or teeth, a nerve block might be required. An infraorbital nerve block will anaesthetise the anterior superior alveolar nerve which innervates

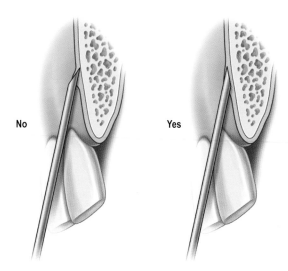

No   Yes

Fig. 4.4   The bevel of the needle should be orientated towards the bone to avoid scraping the periosteum with the sharp tip of the needle.

the anterior maxillary teeth and a posterior superior alveolar nerve block will anaesthetise the maxillary molars.
- Avoid using a standard dental syringe: it is impossible to aspirate using these syringes. Use a conventional syringe with the smallest readily available needle of appropriate length (often a 23G 40-mm needle).

Intraoral infraorbital nerve block

This block provides excellent anaesthesia for pain involving the upper teeth from the midline to the canine or for lacerations involving the upper lip. It also anaesthetises the maxillary premolars and part of the root of the first maxillary molar in about 70% of patients.

The infraorbital foramen can easily be identified using ultrasound to establish its exact position.

Technique

- Locate the infraorbital foramen, which is about 10 mm inferior to the infraorbital notch (the zygomaticomaxillary suture) and about

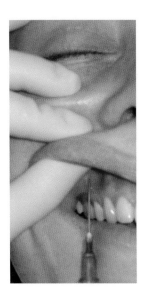

Fig. 4.5 The intraoral approach to the infraorbital nerve block with the needle inserted through the buccal-gingival fold opposite the first premolar and aimed towards a finger palpating the infraorbital foramen.

25 mm lateral to the midline of the face. The patient might experience some discomfort when palpating over the foramen.

- Identify the target area for needle insertion – the apex of the buccal-gingival fold directly adjacent to the first maxillary premolar.
- Dry the mucosa and apply topical anaesthetic.
- Keep your index finger over the infraorbital foramen and lift the lip, pull the tissue taut and shake the lip while inserting the needle, to minimise the pain of injection.
- Keep the syringe parallel to the long axis of the first premolar and direct the needle toward the finger over the infraorbital notch and the infraorbital foramen (Fig. 4.5); keep close to the periosteum to avoid the facial artery.
- Slowly advance the needle until it meets bone (about 10 to 15 mm in an adult), about 10 mm below the inferior orbital margin; do not attempt to enter the infraorbital foramen – this might lead to intraneural injection and further complications.
- Aspirate. If there is no flashback of blood, slowly inject 2 to 5 mL of local anaesthetic.
- If blood is aspirated, withdraw the needle by 5 mm and slightly redirect it while advancing.

- The patient should experience anaesthesia within about 5 minutes of injection.

Posterior superior alveolar nerve block

This nerve block is the preferred alternative to supraperiosteal injection for the maxillary molars when more than two teeth are involved or when infiltration anaesthesia fails or is contraindicated. The block anaesthetises the second and third maxillary molars and, in about 70% of patients, the entire first molar. In the remaining 30% of patients, the posterior superior alveolar nerve innervates all but one root of the first maxillary molar; these patients can be given a supplemental supra-periosteal injection following the block or an infraorbital nerve block if necessary. This block is highly effective but carries a greater risk of intravascular injection and haematoma formation than most other dental blocks. Frequent aspiration is essential during the procedure, so a needle no smaller than 25G is recommended.

Technique

- Identify the target area for needle insertion – the apex of the buccal-gingival fold adjacent to the second maxillary molar.
- Dry the mucosa and apply topical anaesthetic.
- Ask the patient to open their mouth and to move their jaw toward the affected side to create more room.
- Retract the patient's cheek on the side being injected, pull the tissue taut and shake it while inserting the needle.
- Puncture the mucosa at the target area with the syringe aligned with the long axis of the second maxillary molar (Fig. 4.6).

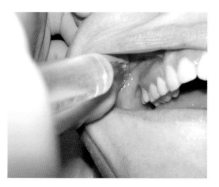

Fig. 4.6 The posterior superior alveolar nerve block is accomplished by firstly puncturing the mucosa of the buccal-gingival fold adjacent to the second molar with the syringe held parallel to the long axis of the tooth. The correct angle of advancement is obtained by moving the syringe in two planes: 45° laterally and then 45° anteriorly (so that the needle is directed medially and posteriorly).

- Advance the needle medially (at a 45° angle) and posteriorly (at a 45° angle to the long axis of the second maxillary molar) to a depth of about 15 mm.
- If bone is contacted, the needle has been directed too medially and should be redirected more laterally.
- Aspirate once, then rotate the syringe by 90° and aspirate again. If there is no flashback of blood, inject 2 to 5 mL of local anaesthetic over 30 to 60 seconds while aspirating periodically during the injection.
- If blood is aspirated, withdraw the needle and redirect it more medially and superiorly.
- Complications (most importantly bleeding) most often result from a needle inserted too deep. If the local anaesthetic was injected with a too shallow needle insertion, adequate anaesthesia may still be attained: too shallow is preferable to too deep with this block.

Local anaesthesia for the mandibular dentition (Fig. 4.7)

Supraperiosteal or infiltration local anaesthesia

This is generally not effective for the mandibular teeth because the thick bony cortex of the mandible is impermeable to local anaesthetic. Nerve block anaesthesia is therefore usually necessary for adequate anaesthesia and analgesia of the lower teeth.

Inferior alveolar nerve block

The inferior alveolar nerve block provides anaesthesia for all the ipsilateral mandibular teeth, the anterior two-thirds of the tongue, and the skin and soft tissue innervated by the mental nerve, and is useful to provide anaesthesia for dental pain and for laceration repair of the anterior tongue and floor of the mouth. The complication rate and failure rate are slightly higher with this block than with some of the other dental blocks. Patients should be warned to avoid self-injury because of the anaesthesia of the lips and tongue.

Technique

- Identify the target area for needle insertion – the area between the pterygomandibular fold and the anterior border of the ramus about 10 mm superior to the occlusal plane of the mandibular teeth (Fig. 4.8).

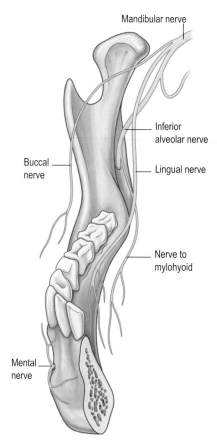

Fig. 4.7 The mandibular nerve and its terminal branches: the auriculotemporal nerve, the long buccal nerve, the mental nerve, the mandibular nerve, the inferior alveolar nerve, and the lingual nerve.

- Apply a topical anaesthetic to this area.
- Insert your thumb into the patient's mouth and place it on the coronoid notch with your index finger just anterior to the ear.
- Retract the cheek laterally to maximise visibility and to decrease the pain of the injection.
- Introduce the needle medial to the centre of your thumb 10 mm above and parallel to the mandibular occlusal plane (Fig. 4.9A).
- Swing the syringe so that the barrel is in the opposite corner of the mouth, resting on the premolars (Fig. 4.9B).

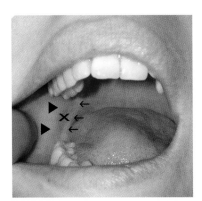

Fig. 4.8 The target area for needle insertion (x) is between the pterygomandibular fold medially (thin arrows) and the anterior margin of the ramus of the mandible laterally (large arrowheads) about 10 mm superior to the mandibular occlusal plane.

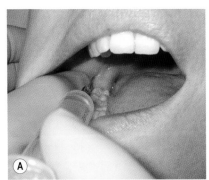

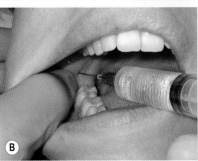

Fig. 4.9 **(A)** The needle is first introduced directly posteriorly until the mucosa is penetrated. **(B)** The syringe is then swung to the opposite side and the needle advanced towards the fingertip that is just anterior to the ear.

- Aim toward your index finger and slowly advance the needle until the bone is contacted, usually a distance of about 25 mm.
- If the needle does not contact bone, redirect the needle more laterally.
- Withdraw the needle 1 mm and aspirate, then rotate the syringe 90° and re-aspirate.
- If there is no flashback of blood, slowly inject 5 mL of local anaesthetic.
- If blood is aspirated, withdraw the needle about 5 mm and reposition it.
- Inject another 2 mL of local anaesthetic while withdrawing the needle.
- If the injection fails to result in adequate analgesia, it can safely be repeated unless the maximum dose of local anaesthetic has been reached.

Intraoral mental nerve block

This is a straightforward, highly successful technique that numbs the mandibular buccal soft tissues from the midline to the second premolar and the skin of the chin and lower lip. It is ideal for patients with trauma to this area who require debridement or laceration repair. The use of a nerve block rather than local infiltration of anaesthetic is particularly advantageous when the laceration involves a cosmetically important structure, such as the vermilion border of the lip, as there is no tissue distortion. The position of the mental foramen is variable but is usually 8 mm superior to the inferior border of the mandible on a line between the premolars or in line with the second premolar; occasionally it is opposite the first molar.

The mental foramen can be identified using ultrasound to establish its exact position.

Technique

- Dry the mucosa and apply topical anaesthetic to the buccal-gingival fold opposite the second premolar.
- Retract, stretch and shake the lower lip to facilitate a painless injection.
- Introduce the needle parallel to the long axis of the second premolar into the target area (Fig. 4.10).
- Advance the needle about 5 mm.

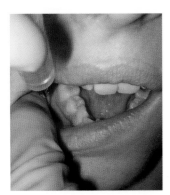

Fig. 4.10 The intraoral mental nerve block is performed with a vertical needle insertion at or slightly posterior to the second premolar. The needle is advanced several millimetres before injecting. A second injection slightly more posterior may be attempted if the initial block is unsuccessful.

- Aspirate. If there is no flashback of blood, slowly inject 5 mL of local anaesthetic.
- If blood is aspirated, withdraw and redirect the needle.
- The patient should experience complete anaesthesia within about 5 minutes of injection.
- If anaesthesia is not successful, reattempt injection slightly posterior to the initial target point.

Lingual nerve block

The lingual nerve supplies sensation to the anterior two-thirds of the tongue and the floor of the mouth. The lingual nerve is often blocked during the inferior alveolar nerve block but may be blocked separately if required. The lingual nerve is a branch of the mandibular nerve and runs in the submucosa medial to the mandibular molars.

Technique

- Identify the target point for needle insertion – the floor of the mouth medial to the third molar.
- Dry the mucosa and apply topical anaesthetic.
- Insert the needle as vertically as possible and advance it about 5 mm (Fig. 4.11).
- Aspirate. If there is no flashback of blood, slowly inject 5 mL of local anaesthetic.
- If blood is aspirated, withdraw and reposition the needle before re-aspirating.

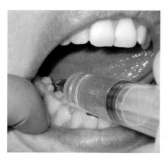

Fig. 4.11 The lingual nerve block can be technically awkward as the tongue may need to be retracted medially. The needle is inserted submucosally opposite the third molar and advanced several millimetres before injecting local anaesthetic.

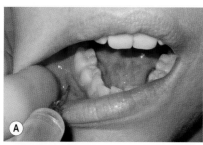

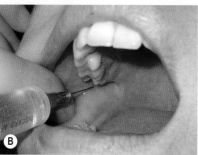

Fig. 4.12 The long buccal nerve may be blocked distally where it runs in the submucosa lateral to the first molar (**A**), or more proximally where it crosses the ramus of the mandible (**B**). In the latter approach, the injection point must be in the maxillary occlusal plane as the nerve is always inferior to this level and gravity will assist in transporting the local anaesthetic to the nerve.

Long buccal nerve block

The long buccal nerve supplies some sensation to the anterior mandibular teeth and an area of the cheek lateral to that supplied by the infraorbital nerve (superior to the labial angle, extending laterally towards the zygoma). It crosses the ramus of the mandible at the level of the maxillary occlusal plane from medial to lateral and runs in the submucosa lateral to the molars.

Technique

- Identify the target point for needle insertion – the buccal-gingival fold lateral to the first molar (Fig. 4.12A).
- Dry the mucosa and apply topical anaesthetic.
- Insert the needle parallel to the long axis of the molar and advance it about 5 mm.
- Aspirate. If there is no flashback of blood, slowly inject 5 mL of local anaesthetic.
- If blood is aspirated, remove the needle and reposition it.

An alternative method is to block the nerve where it crosses the ramus of the mandible (Fig. 4.12B):

- Identify the target point for needle insertion – the pterygomandibular fold at the level of the maxillary occlusal plane.
- Insert the needle and advance it directly posteriorly until the bone is contacted, then withdraw the needle by 1 mm.
- Aspirate. If there is no flashback of blood, slowly inject 5 mL of local anaesthetic.
- If blood is aspirated, withdraw the needle by 5 mm and reposition it.

CHAPTER 5

Intravenous regional anaesthesia (IVRA)

Intravenous regional anaesthesia (IVRA) is a simple and effective regional anaesthesia technique for painful procedures on the forearm, wrist and hand (e.g. for the reduction of a distal radius fracture). IVRA produces anaesthesia by direct diffusion of the local anaesthetic from the veins into the adjacent nerves. The main advantages of this technique are its simplicity and reliability. Its disadvantages are the lack of lasting analgesia (the block resolves almost immediately after the release of the tourniquet), the time required for preparation and performance of the block, and the obligatory delay before the cuff can safely be deflated. It is more effective (with less pain and a better reduction) than a haematoma block for the reduction of distal radius fractures and is somewhat simpler than other regional anaesthesia techniques. IVRA is only appropriate for short procedures of less than 45 minutes before tourniquet discomfort becomes intolerable.

Preparation

- Check the equipment: a proper theatre tourniquet system is ideal but an ordinary blood pressure cuff may be used if an assistant is available to keep it inflated to the correct pressure. Check that the cuff is the correct size required and has no leaks.
- Insert an intravenous line on the uninjured limb and ensure that resuscitation medications and equipment are available.
- Insert a small IV cannula (22G) into the hand of the injured limb, through which the local anaesthetic will be administered.
- Administer procedural sedation if required.
- The patient should be in the supine position with the injured arm elevated for 1 to 2 minutes to achieve passive emptying of the veins.
- Prepare the local anaesthetic agent to the required dilution, and calculate the maximum permissible dose for the patient's body weight and general condition. Use only an intravenous formulation of lidocaine. Bupivacaine and ropivacaine are not suitable agents for IVRA.

Technique

- Place the tourniquet on the arm of the limb to be blocked. Wrap the arm beneath the tourniquet with orthopaedic wool to prevent discomfort and skin damage. Ensure that the tourniquet cannot accidentally deflate, become displaced or open causing a sudden release of local anaesthetic into the circulation. An adhesive bandage wrapped around the cuff will prevent accidental release.
- Apply a 100-mm Esmarch bandage (rubber bandage) to the elevated arm. Always *slightly* stretch the Esmarch bandage before applying the next wrap around the arm (enormous, damaging compression pressures can be generated with overenthusiastic application).
- Inflate the cuff to a pressure of 100 mmHg above the systolic blood pressure, or at least 300 mmHg. If a double cuff is used, inflate the proximal cuff first.
- Inject the local anaesthetic slowly through the IV cannula in the dorsum of the hand.
- Lidocaine is the most commonly used drug for intravenous regional anaesthesia. Either a large volume of dilute solution of local anaesthetic (e.g. 20 to 50 mL of 0.5% lidocaine) or a smaller volume of a concentrated drug (e.g. 12 to 15 mL of 2% lidocaine)

is effective. However, smaller volumes are simpler to use and easier to inject and dilution may not be necessary for the block to function well, as long as complete exsanguination is accomplished.

- The onset of anaesthesia is about 5 minutes.
- After 30–45 minutes most patients become unable to tolerate the pain from the tourniquet. When the discomfort becomes unbearable or additional sedation and analgesics are required, inflate a second cuff distal to the first cuff. The proximal cuff may then be deflated, providing immediate relief of discomfort. If a double cuff system is used, inflate the distal cuff and release the proximal cuff after checking that the distal cuff is correctly inflated. This will provide an additional 15–30 minutes of working time.
- At the end of the procedure it is important to deflate the tourniquet correctly to minimise the risk of systemic local anaesthetic toxicity. If the procedure is completed within 45 minutes after the injection of local anaesthetic, use a two-stage deflation. Deflate the cuff for 10 seconds and immediately reinflate it for 1 minute before the final release. This allows for a more gradual 'washout' of local anaesthetic.
- If the procedure is completed within 20 minutes after injection of local anaesthetic, gradually release the tourniquet in several steps, with 2-minute intervals between deflations.

Complications

- Systemic toxicity of local anaesthetic: The risk mainly comes from an inadequate tourniquet application or equipment failure at the beginning of the procedure; every precaution should be undertaken to ensure that the tourniquet is reliable and the pressure is maintained; gradually release the tourniquet in steps to prevent a massive systemic release of local anaesthetic, especially if the procedure lasts less than 45 minutes.
- Haematoma: Use a small IV catheter; when the superficial veins are punctured during an unsuccessful attempt at placement of the IV catheter, apply firm pressure on the puncture site for 2–3 minutes. Failure to do so will invariably lead to venous bleeding during application of the Esmarch bandage.

The 'Hill block' is a modification of the Bier block for procedures on the wrist and hand. A single cuff tourniquet is placed on the distal forearm, an IV cannula is placed on the dorsum of the hand (facing distally), the limb is exsanguinated and 10 mL of lidocaine 2% is injected for anaesthesia. This technique reportedly causes less tourniquet pain and has fewer complications than the traditional Bier block. Apart from the mentioned differences, the rest of the technique remains the same.

Bier block of lower limb

This is an infrequently used block, but is probably underused as it provides excellent anaesthesia of the foot and is easy to administer. It is performed in exactly the same manner as the block of the upper limb, but an appropriately sized cuff is placed around the ankle and the local anaesthetic is administered into a vein in the dorsum of the foot. The same dose can be used as in the block of the upper limb; the total dose must not exceed the maximum permissible dose based on body weight.

The 'Hill block' is a modification of the Bier block for procedures on the ankle and foot. A single cuff tourniquet is placed on the distal leg, an IV cannula is placed on the dorsum of the foot (facing distally), the limb is exsanguinated and a solution of lidocaine 2% 10 mL plus ketorolac 30 mg (1 mL) is injected for anaesthesia (a lower total dose of anaesthetic is used with this modified method). This technique reportedly causes less tourniquet pain and has fewer complications than the traditional Bier block. Apart from the mentioned differences, the rest of the technique remains the same.

CHAPTER 6

Nerve block regional anaesthesia

General principles

Nerve block regional anaesthesia is potentially of enormous value in the ED. It is useful both for providing an excellent quality of analgesia following traumatic injuries (e.g. a metacarpal block for a crushed finger; a femoral block for a fractured femur; a sciatic nerve block for a fractured ankle) as well as for providing anaesthesia for minor procedures (interscalene block for shoulder dislocation; ankle block for complex wound repair on the foot). There is good evidence to support the efficacy and safety of regional anaesthetic techniques in the ED both in adults and in children.

Some blocks have a high success rate with a blind technique without a nerve stimulator (e.g. femoral block, sciatic block, axillary block, supraclavicular block, interscalene block), but some blocks require a nerve stimulator (e.g. infraclavicular block), and most blocks are probably more successful with the use of nerve stimulators, although this is often debated. The use of ultrasound with or without nerve stimulators can further increase the ease and success rate of nerve plexus or peripheral nerve blockade. There is good clinical evidence to support this, and this is the technique that emergency medicine practitioners should learn and adopt. Studies have shown that ultrasound can decrease the failure rate of nerve blocks from a historical 20–30% to as little as 5% and that the speed of onset can be increased and the complications decreased.

Nerve blocks work on the principle of inducing analgesia or anaesthesia to a body region by injecting a local anaesthetic agent around the nerve or nerves innervating that region. Various techniques may be used to assist in positioning the needle tip adjacent to, but not penetrating, the nerve: the paraesthesia technique; the nerve stimulator; the ultrasound-guided block. Once the needle is located within the neural sheath, a large volume of local anaesthetic is injected (not under pressure) which spreads completely around the nerve (this can also be confirmed with ultrasound). Block success is increased if large volumes are used. Newer evidence with ultrasound-guided blocks shows that smaller volumes can be used because the local anaesthetic can be deposited circumferentially around the nerve under direct vision.

Adverse events following nerve block anaesthesia can include vasovagal reactions, systemic reactions to the local anaesthetic agent (including anaphylaxis, allergic reactions, toxic reactions and methaemoglobinaemia), local tissue pain and inflammation, as well as complications that can vary with the site being punctured. These complications can include nerve damage from intraneural injection, spinal cord damage or total spinal anaesthesia (interscalene block), phrenic or recurrent laryngeal nerve paralysis, pneumothorax or vascular puncture (interscalene or supraclavicular blocks). Fortunately these are rare and can mostly be avoided by meticulous attention to safety and the use of ultrasound techniques.

There are a few important factors to consider before embarking on a nerve block:

- Obtain a focused history from the patient, especially about possible allergies to agents to be used for the procedure contemplated.
- Obtain written consent for the procedure if possible.
- Ensure that there are no contraindications – for example, the interscalene block might not be a good choice for a patient with respiratory compromise.
- Evaluate the general condition of the patient and tailor the procedure and the choice and quantity of medications appropriately.
- Check and document the underlying neurovascular status before commencing with the block: any nerve in the distribution of a

block should be evaluated. Blocks for injuries to the hand should include sensory testing with two-point discrimination (less than 6 mm is normal) in the distribution of each digital nerve that might possibly be injured.

- If applicable, discuss the option of the block with the doctor who will be providing definitive care to the patient (so that he or she is aware that the patient does not have neurological fallout) and make a note in the clinical records.

A detailed discussion of the pharmacokinetics and pharmacodynamics of local anaesthetic agents is beyond the scope of this book. In general, the choice of agents depends on the clinical setting, the required duration of anaesthesia or analgesia, the potential side effects, and, of course, availability. A sound knowledge of the pharmacology of local anaesthetics is not difficult, as there are only a handful of injectable agents readily available. The most commonly used agents for nerve block regional anaesthesia are lidocaine, bupivacaine, mepivacaine and ropivacaine, often with adrenaline (epinephrine) added in a concentration of 1 : 100 000 or lower. Levobupivacaine is a newer formulation, composed exclusively of the S-isomer of bupivacaine (regular bupivacaine is a mixture of the S- and D-isomers). The S-isomer has been shown to be more potent and longer acting, with a more favourable side-effect profile. This agent is much more expensive than the others, however.

The success of the block, the time of onset and the duration of anaesthesia depend on the volume of local anaesthetic agent injected, the agent used and the accuracy of injection. It is important to emphasise that the use of lidocaine in a nerve block does not necessarily accelerate the onset of the block significantly, as part of the lag time results from local tissue diffusion which remains much the same for any agent.

Ultrasound fundamentals for nerve blocks

Conventional peripheral nerve block techniques are performed 'blind', without visual guidance and are completely dependent on surface anatomical landmarks for localisation of nerves or nerve bundles. Some landmark techniques are better than others, since those that rely on bony landmarks have a higher success rate than those using soft-tissue landmarks. Even though the use of nerve stimulators increases the likelihood of placing the needle in proximity to the nerve, needle positioning is still dependent on external or palpable landmarks.

It is, therefore, not surprising that regional anaesthetic techniques have a reported failure rate of up to 20% because of incorrect needle and/or local anaesthetic placement. Multiple trial-and-error attempts at needle placement lead to frustration, unwarranted patient pain and time delay. Ultrasound is a practical option for assisting in nerve blocks as it is portable and non-invasive. ED physicians are also often familiar with ultrasound-guided procedures and can make the transition to ultrasound nerve blocks with ease.

The advantages of ultrasound-guided nerve blocks include the following:

- Nerves can often be clearly visualised on ultrasound. In transverse (cross-sectional) view they appear as round, oval or triangular structures. They are mostly echogenically heterogeneous structures (honeycomb appearance) with hypoechoic predominance (e.g. in the interscalene and supraclavicular regions) or hyperechoic predominance (e.g. in the infraclavicular and popliteal regions).
- Ultrasound shows exactly the nerve location and is especially valuable in patients with anomalous anatomical landmarks. If the nerve itself cannot be visualised, its position can usually be precisely inferred from landmarks and tissue planes visible on ultrasound.
- Ultrasound provides real-time imaging guidance during needle advancement, which allows for continuous adjustments in direction and depth of insertion. This can be done using in-plane or out-of-plane approaches.
- Ultrasound can be used to identify vulnerable structures which might be adjacent to the target nerves, such as blood vessels and the pleura, and enables them to be avoided while still positioning the needle close to the nerve.
- It demonstrates the local anaesthetic spread pattern at the time of injection, and in the case of incomplete spread, the needle can be repositioned under direct vision. At least one repositioning of the needle is normally recommended in any block.
- It improves the quality of sensory block, the onset time and the success rate as compared with the nerve stimulator techniques.
- It may also lessen the number of needle attempts at nerve localisation and potentially reduces the risk of nerve injury, although this has not been proven.

In the real world of the ED, however, visualisation of nerves may not be as easy as described in training material, and the pictures you obtain may not look like those in the book. That does not necessarily reflect on your skill – images in books are always the best available. The images in this book are average images that you might expect to obtain yourself with average equipment. Here are some hints that might help you locate the nerves as easily as possible and how to optimise the imaging capability of your equipment:

- Try to follow the same routine to identify important ultrasound anatomical landmarks – each procedure has certain features that need to be visualised in order to locate the nerves easily. Often these features are blood vessels which can easily be seen with ultrasound, with the assistance of colour Doppler if necessary. Nerves often have a predictable relationship to these vessels.
- Position the probe accurately in the relevant body region according to external landmarks. Ultrasound does not completely eliminate the need for anatomical landmarks.
- Establish the target depth – this is a lot less variable than you might think.
- If you cannot immediately find the nerve, try raising or lowering the frequency of the probe you are using (lower frequency = deeper penetration = less detail; higher frequency = less penetration = greater detail).
- In general, a lower gain is better than a higher setting, as nerves are often subtle shadows and may be obscured in a 'snowstorm' screen.
- Move the focus point or points to the depth of interest (often a bit deeper than the automatic setting).
- Make sure your depth of scan is deep enough to cover the target depth.
- Move the ultrasound probe back and forth over the course of the nerve and look for the honeycomb density of the nerve. Angling the probe may also prove useful – some nerves are visible only when the beam is at 90° to the nerve (anisotropy). Angling back and forth may make the nerve become obvious. Look for contiguous structures that might branch, that remain within the planes between muscles, and that move little with movements of the patient.
- If possible, try repositioning the patient's limb or neck (as appropriate).

- There may be additional presets or adjustments on your machine that might make your life easier – learn to use them.

There are two kinds of needle-to-probe alignments. Each approach has advantages and disadvantages, and some nerve blocks are easier with one than the other. This is covered under the descriptions for each block.

The in-plane approach (Figs 6.1, 6.2A–D)

In this technique the nerve is centred in the display and the needle path is planned – it will enter the field of view from the top right or left. The needle is inserted beneath the long axis of the probe and manoeuvred in line with the ultrasound beam. The advantages of the in-plane approach are that it provides full visualisation of the entire needle shaft and tip when the needle and beam are correctly aligned. This is especially important when there are vital structures in the vicinity of the nerve or in the projected path of the needle (e.g. the supraclavicular block is performed close to the pleura). It also shows the distance between the tip of the needle and the nerve and the movement of the needle towards the target nerve, so that adjustments of angle and direction can be made while advancing the needle.

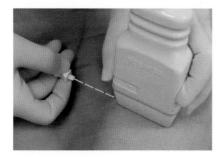

Fig. 6.1 For the in-plane approach, the needle is introduced from the edge of the probe (it does not matter from which edge as long as the operator has the probe orientated correctly) and aligned precisely with the long axis of the probe. Good hand–hand–eye (probe–needle–screen) coordination takes some time to develop. This example shows the probe on the forearm in preparation to perform a radial nerve block just below the elbow via the in-plane approach.

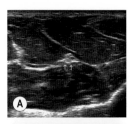
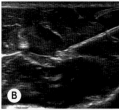
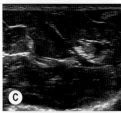
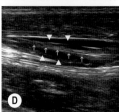

Fig. 6.2 (A) This is the in-plane approach to the median nerve FUN block on the left forearm. The median nerve is visualised in cross-section by placing the probe transversely across the mid-forearm. The nerve is indicated by the arrows. **(B)** The needle has been inserted from the medial aspect of the probe and the tip of the needle can be seen to be positioned immediately superficial to the nerve. This is the main advantage of the in-plane approach: the entire needle can be visualised. **(C)** Local anaesthetic has been injected immediately superficial (anterior) to the nerve and appears as an anechoic area that has distended the tissue around the nerve. As the injection progresses, the local anaesthetic will spread all around the nerve. If necessary, and as is often done routinely, the needle can be repositioned and additional local anaesthetic injected. **(D)** During and after the injection process the circumferential spread of local anaesthetic around the nerve should be confirmed. This can be done using a transverse or longitudinal view of the nerve. For this view the probe is rotated by 90° until an image such as this is obtained. The arrows point to the median nerve in longitudinal view and the arrowheads show the local anaesthetic anterior and posterior to the nerve. This will accurately predict block success.

The disadvantages of the in-plane approach are that it is technically more difficult because it requires accurate alignment of the ultrasound beam with the needle and the nerve. The needle path is not the shortest distance from the skin to the nerve, and the needle often penetrates muscle layers, which might make it more painful. It also requires a needle puncture site which is often different to the traditional nerve-block techniques.

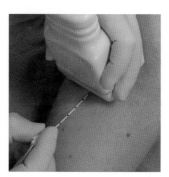

Fig. 6.3 For the out-of-plane approach, the needle is introduced from the long side of the probe closest to the operator. The position of the needle tip can be inferred from local tissue movement and from tissue expansion and the appearance of anechoic local anaesthetic during injection. The needle tip can be seen by sliding the probe away from the operator to locate the tip as the furthest part of the needle that can be visualised. This example shows the probe on the forearm in preparation to perform a radial nerve block just below the elbow via the out-of-plane approach.

Out-of-plane approach (Figs 6.3, 6.4A–E)

In this technique the nerve is centred in the display and the needle path is planned – it will enter from the top of the field of view. The needle is inserted precisely under the centre of the long side of the probe so that the needle and probe are perpendicular to each other. The needle is visualised by ultrasound as a hyperechoic white dot but it can be difficult to identify the tip of the needle. Slide the probe away from the needle puncture site and the hyperechoic dot that is most distant and deep represents the tip of the needle. The advantages of the out-of-plane approach are that this approach resembles the conventional nerve block approach and that by passing the needle perpendicular to the probe the shortest path to the nerve is followed. This is technically easier than the in-plane approach.

The disadvantages are that it can be difficult to accurately localise the needle tip and the needle tip position can only be inferred by observing local tissue movement or tissue expansion at the time of fluid injection.

Optimising the ultrasound image for nerve blocks

The ability to locate and clearly visualise a nerve or group of nerves using ultrasound depends on the emergency physician's knowledge of the relevant surface landmarks, the ultrasound anatomy, the ability to manipulate the probe correctly and the knowledge to optimise the image displayed by the ultrasound machine. The surface and ultrasound anatomy can be learnt from experience and standard teaching material, but the wielding of the wand and the stroking of the machine from experience only.

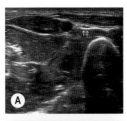

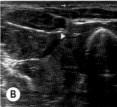

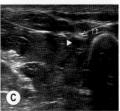

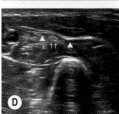

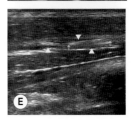

Fig. 6.4 (A) This is the out-of-plane approach to the radial nerve FUN block on the left forearm. The radial nerve is visualised in cross-section by placing the probe transversely across the mid-forearm. The nerve is indicated by the arrows and lies immediately lateral to the radial artery. The nerve is flattened between two fascia layers. **(B)** The needle has been inserted from the centre of the long side of the probe and the tip of the needle can be seen as a small hyperechoic dot (arrow) with an acoustic shadow (arrowhead) and is positioned superficial and slightly medial to the nerve. The path from skin to nerve is much shorter with this approach than with the in-plane approach, but the needle itself is poorly visualised. **(C)** Local anaesthetic has been injected immediately medial to the nerve and appears as an anechoic area (open arrowhead) that has distended the fascial planes around the nerve (arrows) and displaced the nerve laterally. As the injection progresses, the local anaesthetic will spread all around the nerve. If necessary, and as is often done routinely, the needle can be repositioned and additional local anaesthetic injected. The acoustic shadow of the needle is faintly visible (solid arrowhead). **(D)** Local anaesthetic (arrowhead) has spread all around the radial nerve (arrows) and the image of the nerve has become more distinct. **(E)** The longitudinal view of the radial nerve (arrows) confirms anterior and posterior spread of local anaesthetic (arrowhead) and promises a successful block.

The important settings on the machine required for optimum visualisation are:

- *The depth of field.* The depth of field must be adjusted appropriately to match the location of the target of interest. For example, the depth of field should be set within 20 to 30 mm for a superficial structure located 10 mm below the skin surface. There is no set rule, but the size of the target structure should be maximised by selecting an appropriate depth setting.
- *The focus point.* The focus point should be set at or just below the target area of interest.
- *The gain control.* The gain control adjusts the sensitivity of the receivers in the ultrasound probe. Increasing the gain amplifies the overall signal and noise returning to the probe. It does not amplify the strength of the signal emitted by the probe. When the image appears dark, adjust the gain function button to brighten the overall image and the target. The gain should be adjusted to produce an image that is comfortable for the user to interpret. Most machines will have a primary gain control as well as a secondary control (time gain control) that can be used to adjust near gain and far gain. It is possible to fine tune the brightness of the near field and far field separately with these controls.
- *The frequency setting.* The frequency of a multi-frequency transducer can be adjusted to produce an optimum image. The higher frequency range (10–12 MHz range) is best for imaging superficial structures in the near field, and produces the highest definition possible. Higher frequency ultrasound waves do not penetrate far into tissues, however. The mid-range frequency (9–11 MHz range) is best for imaging targets in the mid field. Definition and tissue penetration are both intermediate. The lower frequency range (8–10 MHz range) is best for imaging targets in the far field, but at the expense of definition – a grainy image is often the result.
- *The manufacturer's preset application settings.* A number of manufacturer's preset application settings are available, and these can be tested to see which gives the best visualisation. Do not be put off by the label – the 'breast' preset may give the best image for nerve visualisation in a particular patient. The 'musculoskeletal' preset is generally the best choice, however.
- *Colour Doppler.* Colour Doppler is a useful feature to differentiate a vessel (artery or vein) from a nerve. It is also helpful to locate

vessels that are important landmarks for nerve structures. The colour Doppler function can be used to show vessels in colours which differentiate direction of flow: blue indicates flow away from the probe and red indicates flow towards the probe (BART = blue away, red towards).

Ultrasound probe sterile preparation

For any procedure where the skin is breached (nerve blocks or vascular access) it is important to maintain a sterile field. For this reason, the skin should be cleaned with an appropriate agent (chlorhexidine in 70% alcohol is the most widely used solution) and then draped. Sterile gloves with or without a gown should be used by the operator.

Cover the ultrasound probe with a commercial sterile sheath. If one is not available, simply place a sterile adhesive transparent dressing over the probe surface; another option is to use a sterile glove or a sterilised condom to cover the probe (Fig. 6.5A–C). Make sure that ultrasound gel is layered generously between the probe and the inside of the sheath or glove covering it (for adhesive coverings there is no need to put any gel in between the dressing and the probe surface as long as the contact is smooth without any trapped air or wrinkles).

If necessary, wrap a rubber band, or adhesive tape, around the probe to avoid probe movement inside the sheath during ultrasound scanning. Apply plenty of sterile gel onto the skin surface over the target site to avoid any trapping of air between the probe and skin.

Unless a full-sterile sheath is used, only the probe surface that contacts the patient's skin is sterile, the probe handle and cord are not. Either keep 'one hand clean, one hand dirty', or take great care to handle only the part covered by the sterile dressing (the advantage of using a sterile glove as a covering), or get an assistant to manipulate the probe. A sterile drape can be wrapped around the cord if a commercial probe cover is not used.

Nerve stimulator basic operation

The use of nerve stimulators in regional anaesthesia enables the tip of the needle to be manoeuvred into proximity of the nerve before the injection of local anaesthetics, with a corresponding increase in the success rate of the block procedure.

The basic underlying principle of the nerve stimulator is that the stimulus intensity (current) required to produce a muscle twitch is

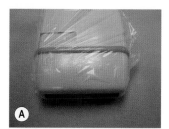

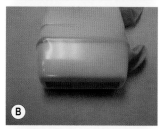

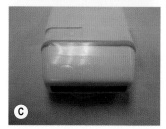

Fig. 6.5 Sterile preparation of the ultrasound transducer may be accomplished using a commercial sterile probe cover or improvised using an adhesive sterile polyurethane dressing **(A)**, a sterile glove **(B)** or a sterilised condom **(C)**.

directly proportional to the distance from the nerve. If the stimulating needle is far from the nerve, a very high stimulus is needed to produce a muscle twitch. Conversely, as the tip moves closer to the nerve a smaller current is required to produce a muscle twitch. With this in mind, once twitches are obtained the current is reduced and the needle manoeuvred until twitches are present at a low current. This indicates proximity of the needle to the nerve. The presence of muscle twitches at very low stimulus intensity, however, raises the concern of intra-neural needle placement.

Use a nerve stimulator that is specifically made for peripheral nerve blocks (not a multifunctional unit, which can be more confusing) with the following characteristics:

- Constant current output. The stimulator automatically compensates for changes in impedance.
- Current meter. The current delivered must be displayed, in units of 0.1 mA.
- Current intensity control. Digital or analogue controlled output.
- Short pulse width. A pulse width of 50 μs to 100 μs is desirable to limit stimulation to α-motor fibres.
- Stimulating frequency. A 2 Hz pulse frequency.
- Disconnect indicator. There might be some other reason for not getting that muscle twitch!

Ensure that you are familiar with the machines that are available to you; it is unlikely that they will be in the ED, but will be available from theatre. Keep current with your techniques and the available technology.

Technique

- Ensure that the negative (black) lead is connected to the needle and that the positive (red) lead is grounded on the patient.
- Set the frequency to 2 Hz, the pulse width to 50 μs, and the initial power output to 0.8 to 1.5 mA (the deeper the nerve, the higher the initial power output – for instance, use 1.5 mA for the sciatic nerve and 0.8 mA for the interscalene block, the axillary block and the femoral block).
- Advance the needle as per the technique for each specific block. As the required twitches are provoked, the current is turned down and the needle carefully advanced until twitches occur at a power output of 0.2 to 0.5 mA. Before injecting, confirm that there are no twitches when the power output is turned below 0.2 mA, as muscle twitches at this power output suggest that the needle tip may be positioned within the nerve.
- Once the position of the needle tip has been confirmed to be close to but not within the nerve, a test dose of 2 to 3 mL of local anaesthetic should be injected. If this dose is sufficient to suppress the motor twitches, this is additional confirmation that the needle tip is appropriately positioned. If this test injection causes severe paraesthesias or severe cramping or aching pain in the distribution of the nerve, this should raise concern about intraneural injection.
- Once the position of the needle has been confirmed with these techniques, then the full volume of the dose may be injected.

CHAPTER 7

Face and neck nerve blocks

Nerve blocks in the head and face are useful for the repair of lacerations and for scrubbing and debriding 'roasties'. Nerve blocks in this region are less painful to the patient than local infiltration and they do not distort the anatomy. The supraorbital nerve, the infraorbital nerve and the mental nerve all exit their foramina along a line that can be drawn 25 mm lateral to the midline of the face through the pupil and the labial angle (Fig. 7.1).

Supraorbital and supratrochlear nerve blocks

The supraorbital and supratrochlear nerves supply sensation to the fontal aspect of the scalp (the forehead). The supraorbital nerve exits the skull through the supraorbital foramen that lies in the midpupillary line, which is approximately 25 mm lateral to the facial midline along the supraorbital ridge. The supratrochlear nerve exits the skull along the upper medial corner of the orbit in the supratrochlear notch, which is approximately 15 mm medial to the supraorbital foramen. Supraorbital and supratrochlear nerve blocks can be performed from either the area of the supraorbital foramen or the area of the supratrochlear notch. When in doubt, an 'eyebrow block' can be used to provide anaesthesia to virtually the entire ipsilateral forehead.

Ultrasound can also be used to identify the precise location of the supraorbital foramen.

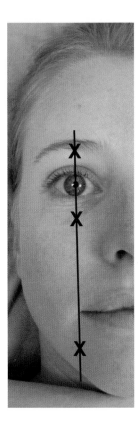

Fig. 7.1 A line drawn through the pupil and the corner of the mouth will bisect the foramina of the supraorbital, infraorbital and mental nerves (from top to bottom).

Technique
Lateral or inferior approach

If performed from the side of the supraorbital foramen (Figs 7.2, 7.3):

- Identify the target area for needle insertion – just lateral to the notch on the supraorbital ridge in the midpupillary line.
- Raise a skin weal of local anaesthetic at the site with a 25G needle.
- Puncture the skin and advance the needle posteriorly and superiorly until the bone is contacted. Withdraw the needle by 1 mm. Do not attempt to enter the foramen.
- Aspirate. If no blood is detected, inject approximately 2 to 3 mL of local anaesthetic outside the foramen above the eyebrow.

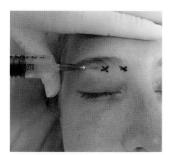

Fig. 7.2 The supraorbital nerve block approached from the lateral side. The needle can be advanced to block the supratrochlear nerve more medially with a single needle insertion.

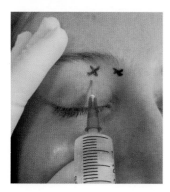

Fig. 7.3 The supraorbital nerve can be blocked from inferiorly. Be careful not to insert the needle into the foramen with this approach. The supratrochlear nerve will need to be blocked with a separate needle insertion.

- If blood is aspirated, reposition the needle slightly and aspirate again.
- If the patient complains of paraesthesias or severe pain with injection, withdraw the needle by 1 to 2 mm before the injection is continued.
- To block the supratrochlear nerve, redirect the needle medially, with the syringe held parallel to the eyebrow, and advance it to a position 15 mm lateral to the junction of the supraorbital ridge and the root of the nose.
- Aspirate. If no blood is withdrawn, inject 1 to 3 mL of local anaesthetic. Inject a further 1 to 3 mL as the needle is withdrawn.

Medial approach

If the block is performed from the area of the supratrochlear nerve (Fig. 7.4):

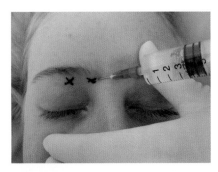

Fig. 7.4 The supratrochlear and supraorbital nerves can be blocked from a medial needle insertion. An 'eyebrow block' will anaesthetise the entire ipsilateral forehead.

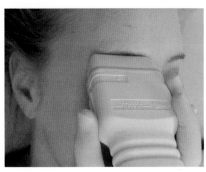

Fig. 7.5 Position the probe just below the eyebrow and angle it posteriorly and superiorly. A conventional probe or, ideally, a small-footprint hockey-stick transducer can be used.

- Identify the target point for needle insertion – the root of the nose at the junction of the nasal root and supraorbital ridge.
- Raise a weal of local anaesthetic at the site with a 25G needle.
- Puncture the skin with the syringe held parallel to the eyebrow. Infiltrate the skin along the length of the entire eyebrow with frequent aspiration to avoid intravascular injection.
- For this field block, 2 to 4 mL of local anaesthetic solution per side is usually sufficient, and no more than 5 mL should be injected into either side.
- Warn patients about the possibility of swelling in the upper and/ or lower eyelids. There is a risk of ecchymosis or haematoma formation with this injection.

Ultrasound assistance

Ultrasound can be used to define the exact position of the supraorbital foramen (Figs 7.5, 7.6A&B). This position can then be marked on the

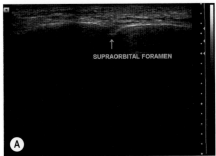

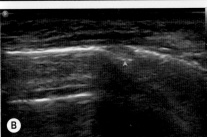

Fig. 7.6 (A)&(B) Ultrasound images showing the 'defect' in the cortex of the supraorbital ridge that indicates the position of the supraorbital nerve foramen (marked by the arrows).

skin and the procedure performed blind (an ultrasound-aided technique) or the out-of-plane approach can be used to advance the needle to a point just superficial to the foramen before injecting local anaesthetic (an ultrasound-guided technique).

Infraorbital nerve block

The infraorbital nerve innervates the lower eyelid, the medial aspect of the cheek, upper lip, and lateral portion of the nose. The infraorbital nerve exits the skull through the infraorbital foramen, which is 10 mm inferior to the orbital rim and approximately 25 mm lateral to the facial midline in the midpupillary line.

An infraorbital block may be performed either via an intraoral approach or by injecting through the skin. *See page 24 in Chapter 4 for the intraoral approach to the infraorbital nerve block.*

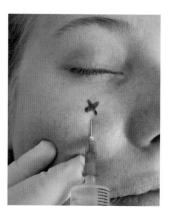

Fig. 7.7 The infraorbital nerve block is performed from inferiorly. Mark the position of the foramen on the skin after palpating it or visualising it with ultrasound.

Technique

Direct transcutaneous injection (Fig. 7.7):

- Identify the target area for needle insertion – 5 mm inferior to the infraorbital foramen.
- Hold the syringe vertically, with the needle aimed superiorly, and puncture the skin 5 mm inferior to the foramen.
- Advance the needle posteriorly and superiorly to contact the bone in the vicinity of the foramen and then withdraw the needle by 1 mm. Do not attempt to enter the canal.
- Aspirate. If no blood is withdrawn, inject 2 to 3 mL of local anaesthetic near and around the foramen, but not into it.
- Keep the injection pressures low since retrograde passage of local anaesthetic into the orbit can cause temporary blindness (very disconcerting to the patient).
- If blood is aspirated, withdraw the needle slightly and redirect it.

Ultrasound assistance

The exact position of this nerve can be more difficult to determine by palpation, but can be easily seen with ultrasound. The probe should be positioned with the edge right against the nose, about 10 mm below the eye (Fig. 7.8). The foramen can be seen as a defect in the cortex (Fig. 7.9A&B). The block can then be performed with real-time ultrasound guidance or once the position has been marked on the skin.

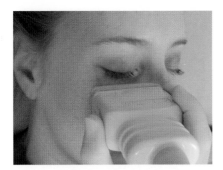

Fig. 7.8 Position the probe just below the eye, abutting against the nose. A normal high-frequency transducer or a hockey-stick type probe can be used.

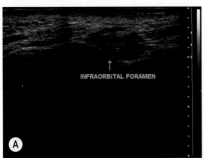

INFRAORBITAL FORAMEN

A

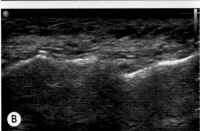

B

Fig. 7.9 (A)&(B) Ultrasound images showing the irregular cortex of the maxillary bone, with the infraorbital foramen marked by arrows.

Mental nerve block

The mental nerve innervates the lower lip and chin. The mental nerve exits the mandible through the mental foramen, which is located approximately 25 mm from the midline of the face in the midpupillary line. Either a transcutaneous or intraoral approach can be used to block the mental nerve. *See page 30 in Chapter 4 for the intraoral approach to the mental nerve block.*

Technique

Direct transcutaneous injection:

- Identify the mental foramen 25 mm lateral to the facial midline, 7 to 10 mm above the inferior border of the mandible.
- This block may be approached from inferiorly (superior needle direction) or from posteriorly (anterior needle direction). The horizontal approach is better if the foramen is not easily palpable, as the position of the foramen can be variable. It is frequently more posterior than expected and a block using this approach will still be successful.
- Posterior approach (Fig. 7.10):
  - The target point for needle insertion is 10 mm posterior to the mental foramen.
  - Hold the syringe parallel to the inferior aspect of the mandible. Puncture the skin 10 mm posterior to the mental foramen and advance the needle into the vicinity of the mental foramen (do not attempt to enter the canal).
  - After aspirating, inject 1 to 2 mL of local anaesthetic near and around the foramen. Inject a further 1 mL while withdrawing the needle. If blood is withdrawn, reposition the needle slightly before injecting.
- Inferior approach (Fig. 7.11):
  - The target point for needle insertion is 5 mm inferior to the mental foramen (immediately superior to the inferior border of the mandible).

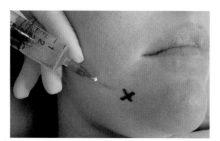

Fig. 7.10 The approach to the mental nerve block from posteriorly increases the chance of block success because local anaesthetic can be deposited to cover a more posterior position of the mental foramen.

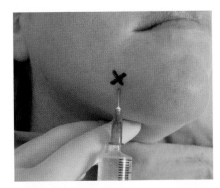

Fig. 7.11 The inferior approach to the mental nerve block. The mental nerve foramen is within 5 to 8 mm of the inferior border of the mandible, so the needle should not be advanced too deep.

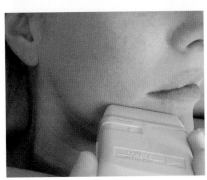

Fig. 7.12 The probe position used to visualise the mental foramen. A small-parts hockey-stick probe, if available, would be a better choice.

- Hold the syringe with the needle pointing superiorly (towards the pupil). Puncture the skin 5 mm inferior to the mental foramen and advance the needle superiorly and posteriorly until the bone is contacted (do not attempt to enter the canal).
- Withdraw the needle by 1 mm and aspirate. If blood is aspirated, reposition the needle slightly.
- If no blood is aspirated, inject 2 to 3 mL of local anaesthetic in the vicinity of the foramen.

Ultrasound assistance

The mental nerve has the most variable bony exit point of the facial nerves. This can be precisely determined using ultrasound (Figs 7.12, 7.13A&B), and the nerve blocked under real-time guidance or blindly after the position has been marked on the skin.

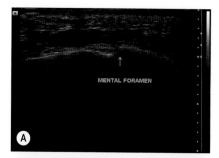

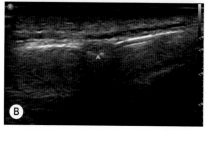

Fig. 7.13 (A)&(B) Ultrasound images of the mandible with the mental foramen clearly visible as an interruption in the cortex (marked by the arrows).

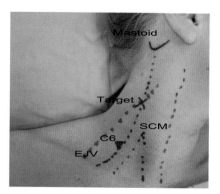

Fig. 7.14 The landmarks for the superficial cervical plexus block. C6, transverse process of C6; EJV, external jugular vein; Mastoid, mastoid process; SCM, sternocleidomastoid muscle with sternal and clavicular heads marked; Target, the midpoint of the line between the mastoid process and the transverse process of C6 at the posterior border of sternocleidomastoid.

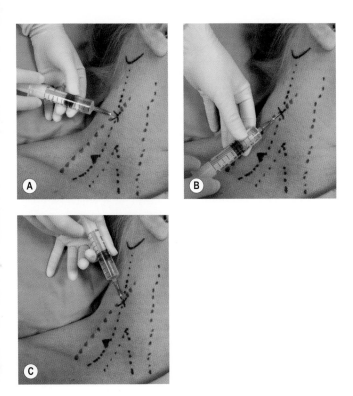

Fig. 7.15 (A)–(C) Local anaesthetic should be infiltrated subcutaneously and just under the lateral margin of sternocleidomastoid 40 mm superior and 40 mm inferior to the midpoint of the line between the mastoid process and the transverse process of C6.

Superficial cervical plexus block

The superficial cervical plexus supplies sensation to the skin of the anterolateral neck through the anterior nerve roots of C2, C3 and C4. This block is useful to provide anaesthesia for procedures or wound repair in the anterior and posterior triangles of the neck.

Preparation

- Position the patient supine or in semi-Fowler's position with the head facing away from the side to be blocked.
- Mark the important landmarks with a skin marker:
  - The mastoid process.
  - The posterior border of sternocleidomastoid (asking the patient to lift their head off the bed tenses the muscle and makes identification easier).
  - The transverse process of C6.
- Draw a line from the mastoid process to the transverse process of C6. Mark the midpoint of this line, which often corresponds to the point at which the external jugular vein crosses the posterior border of sternocleidomastoid. This is the point at which the branches of the superficial cervical plexus emerge from deep to the muscle. This is the target for needle insertion (Fig. 7.14).

Technique

- Prepare the field by cleaning the skin with an antiseptic solution and positioning sterile drapes.
- Identify the target area for the initial needle insertion – the posterior border of sternocleidomastoid at the midpoint of a line connecting the mastoid process to the transverse process of C6.
- Raise a superficial weal of local anaesthetic at the needle insertion site.
- Puncture the skin at the target point with a 25 mm to 50 mm nerve-block needle.
- Inject 10 mL of local anaesthetic subcutaneously along the posterior border of sternocleidomastoid, and just deep to the muscle itself. Use a fan technique to distribute local anaesthetic 30 to 40 mm superior and inferior to the puncture site (Fig. 7.15A–C).
- Avoid deep needle insertion (not more than 10 to 20 mm), and do not advance the needle towards the brachial plexus.
- Subcutaneous midline infiltration of local anaesthetic along a line from the thyroid cartilage to the suprasternal notch will block nerve branches that cross from the contralateral side.
- Aspirate intermittently to avoid intravascular injection.
- Onset of anaesthesia will be within 10 to 20 minutes.

CHAPTER 8

Upper limb blocks

Interscalene block

Use this block for anaesthesia/analgesia of the shoulder joint (dislocation reduction), arm, elbow, and proximal forearm injuries or amputations (Fig. 8.1).

Landmark technique

The interscalene approach to brachial plexus blockade results in anaesthesia of the shoulder, arm, and elbow. It is not consistently reliable for anaesthesia of the hand because the C8 and T1 nerve roots are frequently not blocked, and more distal approaches to the brachial plexus, such as the supraclavicular, infraclavicular or axillary blocks, are more appropriate. The traditional interscalene block relies on the injection and dispersion of a large volume of local anaesthetic within the fascial envelope bordered by the anterior and middle scalene muscles to accomplish blockade of the brachial plexus. This block can be performed at the level of the cricoid cartilage (C6) or slightly more inferiorly, closer to the clavicle. With the more inferior approach, the interscalene groove is shallower and easier to identify and the needle insertion point is much more lateral, which makes vascular puncture rare. This approach is also more suited to those not performing the block regularly.

Preparation

- Position the patient supine or in semi-Fowler's position with the head facing away from the side to be blocked. Position

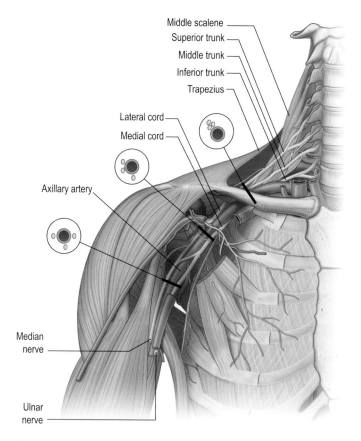

Fig. 8.1 Anatomical diagram of the brachial plexus in the neck and proximal upper limb. The insets show the relative positions of the artery and the nerves in the supraclavicular, infraclavicular and axillary regions as seen on ultrasound.

the patient's arm comfortably by their side and ask them to hold their shoulder down, as though they are reaching for their knee.

- Mark the important landmarks with a skin marker (Fig. 8.2):
  - The clavicle.
  - The cricoid cartilage.

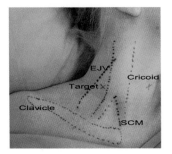

Fig. 8.2 The surface anatomy of the interscalene block is defined by the interscalene groove at the lateral edge of sternocleidomastoid (SCM). The cricoid cartilage (medial X) corresponds with the level of C6 and marks the level of the target for needle puncture (lateral X). The external jugular vein (EJV) should be avoided during needle puncture.

- The posterior border of the clavicular head of the sternocleidomastoid muscle. Ask the patient to turn their head away from the side to be blocked because this tenses the sternocleidomastoid muscles and makes it more prominent. Then ask the patient to lift their head off the table while facing away. This also helps to identify the posterior border of the clavicular head of the sternocleidomastoid muscle.
- The external jugular vein. Ask the patient to try to sit up (or sit forward). This manoeuvre flattens the skin of the neck and helps to identify the interscalene groove, and the Valsalva manoeuvre distends the external jugular vein.
- The interscalene groove. While palpating the posterior border of sternocleidomastoid, ask the patient to forcefully sniff. This tenses the scalene muscles and the interscalene groove becomes more prominent.

Technique
- Prepare the field by cleaning the skin with an antiseptic solution and positioning sterile drapes.
- Identify the target area for the initial needle insertion – the interscalene groove, at about the level of the cricoid cartilage, or slightly inferiorly. The most common error is inserting the needle too far anteriorly. Examine the anatomical landmarks carefully.
- Raise a superficial weal of local anaesthetic at the needle insertion site.
- Puncture the skin at the target point with a 25 mm to 50 mm nerve-block needle (Fig. 8.3A–C). Direct the needle perpendicular to the skin surface – slightly medially, inferiorly 30° to 45° and

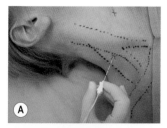

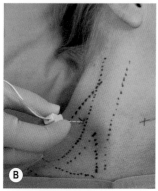

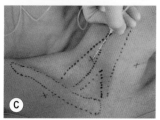

Fig. 8.3 There are many descriptions of the technique for the interscalene block with regards to the location of the puncture site and the angle of needle advancement. Most techniques are equally effective but the incidence of undesirable effects (pneumothorax, vascular puncture and phrenic nerve blockade) has been claimed to be lower with some techniques (such as the 'plumb-bob' technique) than with others. **(A)** The most classical technique: puncture at the level of the cricoid cartilage with needle advancement posteriorly, slightly inferiorly and slightly medially. **(B)** One of the 'plumb-bob' techniques, with puncture at the level of the cricoid cartilage and needle advancement directly posteriorly. **(C)** A technique using the same puncture site, but needle advancement 45° posteriorly towards the centre-point of a line between the jugular fossa and the acromion.

posteriorly aiming at the transverse process of C6. If you are using a more inferior puncture site (25 mm above the clavicle), insert the needle perpendicular to the skin surface taking care not to aim superiorly. The inferior angle of the needle is important to decrease the risk of inadvertent entry into one of the neural foramina.

- Advance the needle 10 to 20 mm until paraesthesias are elicited.

- An alternative method is to use a parasagittal approach with the needle held parallel to the scalene muscles and aimed inferiorly towards the midpoint of the clavicle.
- If you are using a nerve stimulator, insert the needle using the same technique. Appropriate twitches include pectoralis, deltoid, triceps, biceps or any muscle of hand or forearm, but not the trapezius.
- Aspirate. If no flashback of blood is obtained, inject 30 to 40 mL of local anaesthetic slowly with intermittent aspiration to rule out intravascular injection. Slow injection increases block success and decreases complications. If resistance to injection, severe paraesthesias or cramping pain sensations occur with initial injection, then the needle should be withdrawn by 1 to 2 mm to avoid intraneural injection. Use the higher end of the volume range if C8/T1 anaesthesia is desired (remembering that larger volumes are associated with more undesirable effects for this particular block).
- The onset of anaesthesia with lidocaine is from 5 to 15 minutes and with bupivacaine is from 10 to 20 minutes; duration of anaesthesia is 3 to 6 hours and 8 to 10 hours, respectively; duration of analgesia is 5 to 8 hours and 16 to 18 hours, respectively.

Precautions

The interscalene block is very safe if used appropriately and carefully. Avoid using this block in patients who have significant chronic respiratory disease or patients with respiratory distress, as well as in patients with contralateral phrenic nerve or recurrent laryngeal nerve paralysis.

Complications

- Inadvertent total spinal anaesthesia is a potentially serious complication resulting from incorrect needle placement or from local anaesthetic tracking proximally within the nerve root sheath.
- Vertebral artery injection can result in a rapid onset of central nervous system toxicity.
- Phrenic nerve block occurs frequently, so do not use this block bilaterally or in patients with respiratory compromise.
- Recurrent laryngeal, vagus, and cervical sympathetic nerves are often blocked.

- Pneumothorax can occur as the cupola of the lung may be pierced by a poorly directed needle.

Ultrasound technique

This technique is a simple, easy-to-use method, does not require a nerve stimulator, and allows for smaller volumes of local anaesthetic to be used. It allows precise visualisation of the significant structures and avoids misadventures from misplacement of the needle. It is a useful technique for the ED.

Preparation

- Position the patient supine or in semi-Fowler's position with the head facing away from the side to be blocked.
- Rest the arm comfortably by the patient's side or across the abdomen.
- Use a linear high-frequency probe (10 to 15 MHz is ideal) and select an appropriate pre-set application.
- Identify the area to begin the scan – either the midline of the neck or the supraclavicular fossa, depending upon which scan strategy is employed (Fig. 8.4).
- Perform a preliminary non-sterile survey scan to identify the relevant anatomy and optimise the image by adjusting depth of field (about 20 to 30 mm), focus point, and gain. Mark the best probe position on the skin with a pen, if required.
  - Place the probe transversely in the midline at the level of the cricoid cartilage. Move the probe laterally to identify the

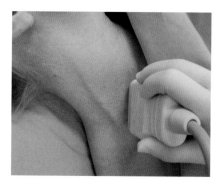

Fig. 8.4 The scan for the interscalene block can be started in the midline and the probe moved laterally to identify the interscalene groove and the brachial plexus, or started in the supraclavicular fossa and the probe moved superiorly while tracing the brachial plexus. The probe can be angled and aligned in order to visualise the nerves optimally.

carotid artery, internal jugular vein and the anterior scalene muscle immediately lateral to the vessels. The brachial plexus can be identified in transverse section in the space between the anterior and middle scalene muscles. In the interscalene region the brachial plexus nerve roots appear as a cluster of round or oval hypoechoic structures (Fig. 8.5A–C).

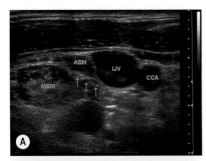

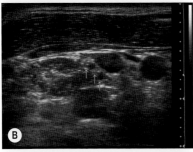

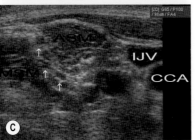

Fig. 8.5 The interscalene groove is located between the middle scalene muscle (MSM) and the anterior scalene muscle (ASM), which are just lateral to the internal jugular vein (IJV) and common carotid artery (CCA). **(A)** The hypoechoic nerve roots are indicated by the arrows. **(B)** The brachial plexus slightly more inferiorly in the interscalene groove. **(C)** The appearance of the hypoechoic nerve roots in a different patient. The brachial plexus can be seen to lie very superficially in the neck – between 10 and 20 mm deep in these images. The site for needle insertion can be selected at any point that is convenient for visualising the nerve roots, with a needle track that is clear of vessels.

- Alternatively, place the probe transversely in the supraclavicular fossa to identify the nerves clustered around the subclavian artery as a 'bunch of grapes'. Then move the probe superiorly to trace the nerves more proximally into the neck.
- Prepare the field by cleaning the skin with an antiseptic solution and positioning sterile drapes. Cover the probe with a sterile probe-sheath and apply sterile ultrasound gel to the area of the interscalene groove.

Technique

In-plane approach (Fig. 8.6)

- Identify the hypoechoic nerve roots in their transverse axis in an area convenient to block.
- Raise a weal of local anaesthetic at the needle insertion target with a 27G needle.
- Insert a 25 mm to 50 mm 22G nerve-block needle on the lateral end of the ultrasound probe.
- Advance the needle towards the edge of the nerves while visualising the entire length of the needle in real time.
- Aim to contact nerve roots in the centre of the interscalene groove from the lateral side; avoid injection close to the neural foramina.
- Track real-time needle movement to prevent inadvertent entry through the neural foramina.

Out-of-plane approach (Fig. 8.7A&B)

- Identify the hypoechoic nerve roots in their transverse axis in an area convenient to block.

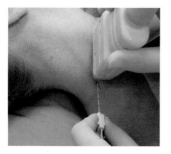

Fig. 8.6 The in-plane approach to the interscalene brachial plexus block is performed from the lateral edge of the probe and the needle is advanced through the middle scalene muscle to the edge of the nerve roots.

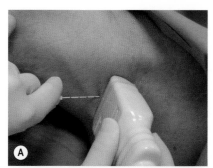

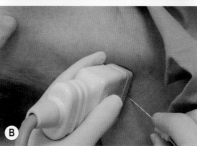

Fig. 8.7 (A)&(B) The out-of-plane approach to the interscalene block may be performed from either side of the probe. The needle position must be carefully assessed during advancement to ensure accurate placement adjacent to the nerve roots.

- Line up the nerve target at the midpoint of the screen. The needle insertion point will correspond to the exact centre of the transducer.
- Raise a weal of local anaesthetic at the needle insertion target with a 27G needle.
- Insert a 25 mm to 50 mm 22G nerve-block needle on the superior or inferior side of the ultrasound probe.
- Observe tissue and needle movement as the needle is advanced towards the target. Aiming for the side of the nerve bundle rather than the centre makes needle placement more accurate.
- Clear identification of the needle tip may require the probe to be angled back and forth.

The injection process

- Slowly inject local anaesthetic around the nerve roots by positioning the needle in the centre of the interscalene groove, adjacent to the nerve sheath. Aspirate frequently to avoid inadvertent intravascular injection. If resistance to injection, severe paraesthesias or severe cramping pain are provoked in the limb during injection, immediately withdraw the needle by 1 to 2 mm to avoid intraneural injection.

- Observe the local anaesthetic spread during injection. A hypoechoic collection will appear adjacent to and then spread around the nerves.
- An expansion of the tissue in the interscalene groove indicates a correct positioning of the local anaesthetic injection; expansion within the scalene muscle indicates intramuscular injection and the needle should be repositioned.
- Reposition the needle at least once to ensure complete circumferential local anaesthetic spread around the nerve roots.
- The volume of local anaesthesia introduced appears to be directly related to side effects and complications of the interscalene block. Phrenic nerve blockade is more frequent when volumes greater than 10 mL are injected. The use of ultrasound allows for smaller volumes to be placed accurately and effectively. Inject 10 mL of local anaesthetic or just enough that the nerve roots are visualised to be completely surrounded by hypoechoic fluid. Injection of as little as 5 mL of local anaesthetic within (rather than around) the nerve sheath itself can produce an effective block.

Supraclavicular block

Landmark technique

The supraclavicular block is performed below the level of the nerve roots at a point where the brachial plexus trunks have formed and are contained within a neural sheath. This approach produces a rapid-onset block with a predictable, dense anaesthesia. The supraclavicular block can be used to provide anaesthesia and analgesia for the upper limb distal to the shoulder.

Preparation

- Position the patient supine or in semi-Fowler's position with the head facing away from the side to be blocked. Rest the patient's arm comfortably across their abdomen.
- Mark the important landmarks with a skin marker (Fig. 8.8):
  - The posterior border of the clavicular head of the sternocleidomastoid muscle at the point of insertion onto the

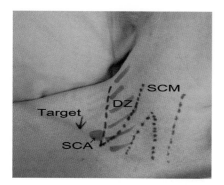

Fig. 8.8 The surface landmarks for the supraclavicular approach to the brachial plexus block. A parasagittal line drawn through the posterior clavicular attachment of sternocleidomastoid (SCM) marks a danger zone (DZ) in which the cupola of the lung extends into the neck. The target point for needle insertion is immediately superior to the clavicle, about 25 mm lateral to the danger area and immediately lateral (posterior) to the pulsation of the subclavian artery (SCA).

clavicle (ask the patient to lift their head off the table while facing away, as this helps to define this landmark).

- Draw a line on the neck parallel to the midline through this point to demarcate the lateral extension of the cupola of the lung. The area medial to this line is a danger area because of the risk of pneumothorax.
- The point of pulsation of the subclavian artery should be marked.
- The target point for needle insertion is approximately 25 mm lateral to the line (as a margin of safety) and should be marked on the skin.

Technique

- Prepare the field by cleaning the skin with an antiseptic solution and positioning sterile drapes.
- Identify the target area for needle insertion – about 25 mm lateral to the posterior border of sternocleidomastoid and 15 mm (one fingerbreadth) superior to the clavicle. This should be immediately posterolateral to the pulsation of the subclavian artery superior to the clavicle.
- Raise a superficial weal of local anaesthetic at the needle insertion site with a 27G needle.
- Puncture the skin at the target point with a 25 mm to 50 mm nerve-block needle. Insert the needle perpendicularly to the skin and advance it 2 to 5 mm (Fig. 8.9A&B). Redirect the needle inferiorly, keeping it parallel to the scalene muscles (in a slightly lateral direction) until paraesthesias are elicited. The insertion

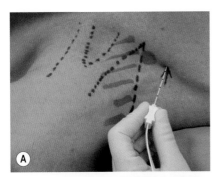

Fig. 8.9 (A) The supraclavicular block is performed by advancing the needle towards the first rib from just lateral to the subclavian artery. The needle should be kept parallel to the scalene muscles or slightly laterally directed. An alternative method **(B)** is to advance the needle directly posteriorly from the insertion point until the brachial plexus is contacted.

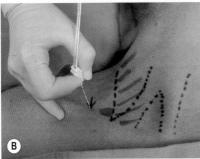

depth is unlikely to be more than 25 mm. Once the rib is contacted the needle can be 'walked' anteriorly and posteriorly while keeping the syringe parallel to the interscalene groove until the brachial plexus is located. If the rib is not found, the needle should be carefully redirected first laterally and then medially until it is contacted or paraesthesias or nerve twitches are elicited.

- If you are using a nerve stimulator, insert the needle using the same technique. The needle is advanced slowly until flexion or extension twitches of the fingers are obtained.
- Aspirate. If no flashback of blood is obtained, inject 30 to 40 mL of local anaesthetic slowly with intermittent aspiration to rule out intravascular injection. Slow injection increases block success and decreases complications. If resistance to injection, severe paraesthesias or cramping pain sensations occur with initial injection, the needle should be withdrawn by 1 to 2 mm to avoid intraneural injection.

- The onset of anaesthesia with lidocaine is from 5 to 15 minutes and with bupivacaine is from 10 to 20 minutes; duration of anaesthesia is 3 to 6 hours and 8 to 10 hours, respectively; duration of analgesia is 5 to 8 hours and 16 to 18 hours, respectively.

Precautions

This block is very safe if used appropriately and carefully. Avoid using this block in patients who have significant chronic respiratory disease or patients with respiratory distress, as well as in patients with contra-lateral phrenic nerve or recurrent laryngeal nerve paralysis.

Complications

Common side effects associated with this technique include phrenic nerve block with diaphragmatic paralysis and sympathetic nerve block with development of Horner's syndrome. This usually only requires reassurance for the patient. Phrenic nerve block occurs in about 50% of cases and is not associated with respiratory dysfunction in healthy volunteers.

Pneumothorax associated with supraclavicular block is not common, is generally small requiring conservative treatment only, and develops within a few hours following the procedure. In rare instances its presentation can be delayed up to 12 hours.

Complications similar to those occurring with other peripheral blocks, such as intravascular injection with development of systemic local anaesthetic toxicity, as well as haematoma formation, may occur. Neurapraxias and neurologic injury are similarly possible, but rarely reported.

Ultrasound technique

This technique is a simple, easy-to-use method, does not require a nerve stimulator, and allows for smaller volumes of local anaesthetic to be used. It also virtually abolishes the likelihood of inadvertent vascular and pleural puncture.

Preparation

- Position the patient supine or in semi-Fowler's position with the head facing away from the side to be blocked.
- Rest the arm comfortably by the patient's side or across the abdomen.

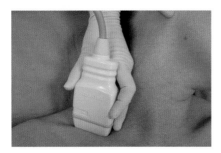

Fig. 8.10 The ultrasound probe is positioned just superior to the clavicle for the supraclavicular block. The probe must be angled posteriorly and inferiorly to first locate the subclavian artery, which is the major landmark for the block. The nerves will be found lateral and superficial to the subclavian artery and are usually easily visible.

- Use a linear high-frequency probe (10 to 15 MHz is ideal) and select an appropriate pre-set application.
- Identify the area to begin the scan – either the midline of the neck or the supraclavicular fossa.
- Perform a preliminary non-sterile survey scan to identify the relevant anatomy and optimise the image by adjusting depth of field (20 to 30 mm), focus point, and gain. Mark the best probe position on the skin with a pen, if required. Position the probe over the supraclavicular fossa in the transverse plane to obtain the best possible cross-sectional view of the subclavian artery and brachial plexus (Figs 8.10, 8.11A–C). Scan proximally and distally to observe the nerve roots and nerve trunks. The nerves in this region are round or oval, are hypoechoic, and can be found lateral and superficial to the subclavian artery (which can be identified with the assistance of colour Doppler if necessary) and superior to the first rib. The subclavian vein is medial to the artery. Visualise the pleura (check for the pleural sliding sign and comet tails) and note the relation to the brachial plexus and the planned needle track. Also take note of the distance from the skin to the rib and the skin-to-pleura distance.
- Prepare the field by cleaning the skin with an antiseptic solution and positioning sterile drapes. Cover the probe with a sterile probe-sheath and apply sterile ultrasound gel to the area of the supraclavicular fossa.

Technique

In-plane approach (lateral to medial)

This approach is considerably different from the conventional supra-clavicular techniques. The block needle is inserted in a very lateral

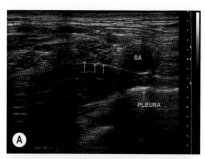

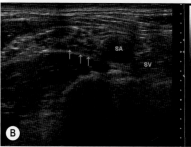

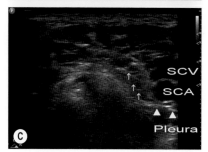

Fig. 8.11 **(A)–(C)** The subclavian artery (SA/SCA) lies lateral (or occasionally deep) to the subclavian vein (SV/SCV) and close to the pleura. The brachial plexus nerves are lateral to the artery and readily accessible for blocking under real-time ultrasound guidance. If the nerves are not easily visible, the artery can be used as a guiding landmark to position the needle.

position and advanced in a lateral to medial direction starting from the lateral edge of the probe. The in-plane approach enables the physician to track the needle tip in real time in order to minimise the risk of accidental pleural or vascular puncture.

- Identify the hypoechoic nerve roots in their transverse axis in the supraclavicular fossa.

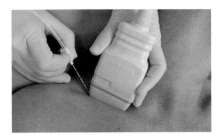

Fig. 8.12 Once the optimum image has been obtained the needle is inserted at the lateral end of the probe and advanced towards the lateral edge of the brachial plexus nerves under direct ultrasound visualisation.

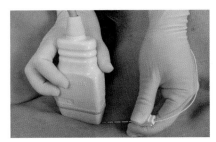

Fig. 8.13 The in-plane approach, which makes use of a medial needle insertion, may be suitable if the nerves lie predominantly superficial to the artery.

- Raise a weal of local anaesthetic at the needle insertion target with a 27G needle.
- Insert a 25 mm to 50 mm 22G nerve-block needle on the lateral end of the ultrasound probe.
- Advance the needle towards the edge of the nerve bundle while visualising the entire length of the needle in real time and avoiding pleural or vascular puncture (Fig. 8.12).

An alternative in-plane approach (medial to lateral)

The advantage of ultrasound guidance is that any approach can be used and the needle tip can be positioned next to the nerves under direct vision (Fig. 8.13). While this approach has the advantage of advancing the needle away from the artery and the pleura, it also makes it more difficult to position the needle close to the nerves if they lie deep or directly lateral to the artery.

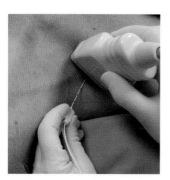

Fig. 8.14 The out-of-plane approach is favoured by many clinicians for this block, despite the proximity to the pleura. This is because of the shorter skin-to-nerve distance and the similarity to the traditional landmark technique.

Out-of-plane approach

This is similar to the traditional blind landmark approach. The needle is introduced and advanced into the proximity of the nerve (Fig. 8.14).

* Identify the subclavian artery and the round hypoechoic nerve trunks of the brachial plexus located lateral to the artery, with the probe in the transverse plane in the supraclavicular fossa.
* Raise a weal of local anaesthetic with a 27G needle at the needle insertion point on the superior side of the transducer.
* Introduce a 25 mm to 50 mm 22G nerve-block needle perpendicular to the superior aspect of the probe.
* Advance the needle carefully towards the edge of the nerve trunks. While the needle itself might not be visible, its progress can be assessed by local tissue movement and the tip can be followed by angling the probe back and forth in order to avoid pleural or vascular puncture.

The injection process

* Slowly inject local anaesthetic around the nerve roots by positioning the needle adjacent to the nerve sheath. Aspirate frequently to avoid inadvertent intravascular injection. If resistance to injection, severe paraesthesias or severe cramping pain are provoked in the limb during injection, immediately withdraw the needle by 1 to 2 mm to avoid intraneural injection.
* Observe the local anaesthetic spread during injection. A hypoechoic collection will appear adjacent to and then spread around the nerves. If no fluid collection develops, then ensure that intravascular injection has not occurred.

- Observe the pattern of local anaesthetic spread around the target nerves during injection. Inject most of the local anaesthetic immediately superior to the first rib and next to the subclavian artery if anaesthesia to the distal forearm and hand is desired, because the ulnar nerve often lies in this position, posterior to the subclavian artery.
- Reposition the needle at least once to ensure complete circumferential local anaesthetic spread around the nerve roots.

Infraclavicular block

Landmark technique

The infraclavicular block is a blockade of the brachial plexus in the region of the coracoid process. This provides good anaesthesia for the hand, wrist, forearm, elbow, and distal arm, but is not a good choice for anaesthesia or analgesia for the shoulder, the axilla and the proximal medial arm. The coverage is similar to that of the supraclavicular block.

This block may be the one of most useful of the brachial plexus blocks in the acute trauma patient when there is limited access to the neck and it is an advantage not to have to move the limb to allow the block to be administered.

Preparation

- Position the patient supine with the head facing away from the side to be blocked.
- The arm can be kept at the patient's side or across their abdomen, but ideally the arm should be abducted at the shoulder and flexed at the elbow to keep the relationship of the landmarks to the brachial plexus constant. Make sure that you can visualise the twitches of the hand.
- With a pen, mark the important landmarks for the infraclavicular block (Fig. 8.15):
  - The medial end of clavicle.
  - The coracoid process – as the arm is elevated and lowered the coracoid process can be felt medial to the shoulder.
  - The midpoint of a line connecting the medial end of clavicle and the coracoid.
  - The needle insertion point – 30 mm inferior and perpendicular to the midpoint of the line between the medial end of the clavicle and the coracoid.

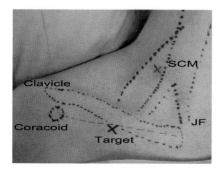

Fig. 8.15 The surface anatomy for the infraclavicular block. The target point for needle insertion is the midpoint of a line between the medial end of the clavicle and the coracoid process, immediately inferior to the clavicle. JF, jugular fossa; SCM, sternocleidomastoid.

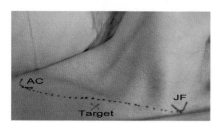

Fig. 8.16 The surface anatomy for the mid-clavicular vertical needle (or 'plumb-bob') technique. The target point for needle insertion is the midpoint of a line between the jugular fossa (JF) and the most inferior part of the acromion (AC), immediately inferior to the clavicle.

- For the mid-clavicular 'vertical needle' approach, mark the following landmarks (Fig. 8.16):
  - The jugular fossa (suprasternal fossa).
  - The most anterior part of the acromion.
  - The midpoint of a line connecting the jugular fossa and the acromion.
  - The needle insertion point – immediately inferior to the clavicle at the midpoint of the line between the jugular fossa and the acromion. This should be exactly one fingerbreadth (10 mm) medial to the infraclavicular fossa.
- For the sub-coracoid 'vertical needle' approach, mark the following landmarks (Fig. 8.17):
  - The coracoid process.
  - A point 20 mm inferior and 20 mm medial to the coracoid process.

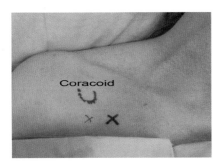

Fig. 8.17 The surface anatomy for the sub-coracoid vertical needle (or 'plumb-bob') technique. The target point for needle insertion is 20 mm inferior and 20 mm medial to the coracoid process.

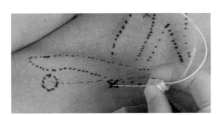

Fig. 8.18 The puncture site is at the midpoint of a line connecting the medial end of the clavicle with the coracoid. The needle is advanced towards the coracoid at a 45° posterior angle until paraesthesias or muscle twitches are produced.

Technique

- Prepare the field by cleaning the skin with an antiseptic solution and positioning sterile drapes.
- Identify the target area for needle insertion – about 30 mm inferior to the midpoint of a line joining the medial end of the clavicle and the coracoid process.
- Raise a superficial weal of local anaesthetic at the needle insertion site with a 27G needle.
- Puncture the skin at the target point with a 100 mm nerve-block needle. Advance the needle laterally at a 45° angle to the skin, parallel to the line connecting the medial clavicular head with the coracoid process (Fig. 8.18).
- The brachial plexus is normally encountered at a needle depth 50 to 80 mm. If paraesthesias or appropriate muscle twitches are not obtained, angle the needle more inferiorly away from the clavicle.
- Twitches from the pectoralis, biceps or deltoid muscles are not necessarily indicative of proximity to the brachial plexus trunks since the musculocutaneous and axillary nerves may depart the nerve sheath more proximally.

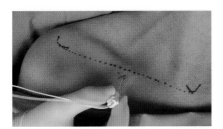

Fig. 8.19 For the mid-clavicular vertical needle technique, the needle is advanced directly posteriorly from a puncture site at the midpoint of a line between the jugular fossa and the inferior tip of the acromion.

- Aspirate. If no flashback of blood is obtained, inject 30 to 40 mL of local anaesthetic slowly with intermittent aspiration to rule out intravascular injection. Slow injection increases block success and decreases complications. If resistance to injection, severe paraesthesias or cramping pain sensations occur with initial injection, the needle should be withdrawn by 1 to 2 mm to avoid intraneural injection.
- *The mid-clavicular vertical needle technique* (Fig. 8.19): Puncture the skin at the target point (immediately inferior to the clavicle at the midpoint of a line joining the jugular fossa and the acromion) with a 50 mm to 75 mm nerve-block needle positioned vertically (not perpendicular to the skin, but truly vertical). Advance the needle directly posteriorly until paraesthesias or appropriate nerve twitches are elicited. Avoid medial direction of the needle as this may result in vascular or pleural puncture. The brachial plexus is seldom deeper than 50 mm from the skin surface even in very large patients, and a penetration depth of greater than 60 mm increases the risk of complications.
- *The sub-coracoid vertical needle technique* (Fig. 8.20): The puncture site is 20 mm inferior and 20 mm medial to the coracoid process. This point is lateral to the ribs (and therefore the lung) and a needle advanced directly posteriorly should pass in proximity to the nerves at a depth of 50 to 100 mm. If no paraesthesias (or muscle twitches) are obtained before the scapula is contacted, the needle should be withdrawn and directed slightly inferiorly. This technique has the advantages of being simple, safe and reliable.

Ultrasound technique

In the vicinity of the coracoid process (the infraclavicular region) the trunks of the brachial plexus are arranged around the axillary artery.

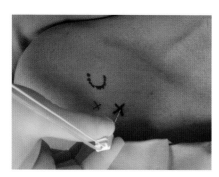

Fig. 8.20 For the sub-coracoid vertical needle technique, the needle is advanced directly posteriorly from the puncture site inferomedial to the coracoid process.

The trunks lie predominantly superiorly and posteriorly to the axillary artery. Since the trunks lie deeply under the skin surface, this block may work with a lower-frequency curvilinear probe.

Preparation

* Position the patient supine with the head facing away from the side to be blocked.
* Rest the arm comfortably by the patient's side or across the abdomen.
* Use a linear high-frequency probe (10 to 15 MHz is ideal) or a curvilinear probe (2 to 6 MHz) and select an appropriate pre-set application.
* Identify the area to begin the scan – the chest wall just below the clavicle and immediately medial to the coracoid process. Perform a preliminary non-sterile survey scan to identify the relevant anatomy and optimise the image by adjusting depth of field (40 to 60 mm), focus point, and gain. Position the probe in the longitudinal plane to visualise the brachial plexus and axillary vessels in a cross-sectional view (Figs 8.21, 8.22A–C). Nerves in this region are normally hyperechoic. The lateral cord is most commonly superior to the axillary artery (9 o'clock position) and the posterior cord posterior to the artery (6 o'clock). When visible, the medial cord is inferior to the artery (3–6 o'clock). Mark the best probe position on the skin with a pen, if required.
* Prepare the field by cleaning the skin with an antiseptic solution and positioning sterile drapes. Cover the probe with a sterile probe-sheath and apply sterile ultrasound gel to the area of the coracoid process.

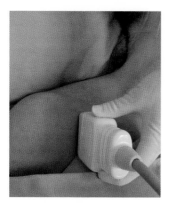

Fig. 8.21 Position the probe in the longitudinal plane immediately medial to the coracoid process. The first landmark is the axillary artery. The artery is surrounded by the nerves superiorly, posteriorly and inferiorly.

Technique

In-plane approach (superior to inferior direction) (Fig. 8.23)

- Identify the hyperechoic nerve roots in their transverse axis in the infraclavicular region and plan the approach.
- Raise a weal of local anaesthetic at the needle insertion target with a 27G needle.
- Insert a 50 mm to 75 mm 20G nerve-block needle at the superior end of the ultrasound probe. A thicker needle is better because it is easier to see on ultrasound with deeper penetration, and because it is deflected less during deep tissue penetration and therefore easier to control.
- Advance the needle at a 45° to 60° angle posteriorly and inferiorly towards the edge of the nerve bundle while visualising the entire length of the needle in real time to avoid pleural or vascular puncture.
- Aim to direct the needle so that local anaesthetic can be injected posterior and superior to the axillary artery.

Out-of-plane approach (Fig. 8.24)

- Identify the hyperechoic nerve roots in their transverse axis in the infraclavicular region and plan the approach.
- Raise a weal of local anaesthetic at the needle insertion target with a 27G needle.

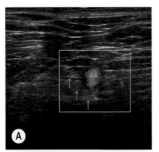

Fig. 8.22 (A)–(C) The axillary artery is easily visible and may be distinguished from the vein using colour Doppler (if necessary). The nerves can usually be seen surrounding the artery, and local anaesthetic should be injected posteriorly and superiorly to the artery to accomplish the block.

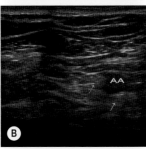

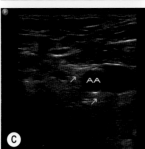

- Insert a 50 mm to 75 mm 20G nerve-block needle at the medial side of the ultrasound probe. Line up the nerve target at the midpoint of the screen and then insert the block needle aligned with the centre of the probe.
- Advance the needle, as with the landmark technique, from medial to lateral at a 45° angle to the skin. The passage of the needle can be inferred from local tissue movement.

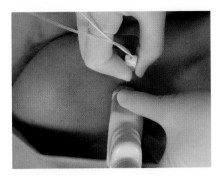

Fig. 8.23 The in-plane approach for the infraclavicular block is performed from the superior edge of the probe. The needle is angled fairly steeply posteriorly and guided to the posterior as well as the superior aspect of the axillary artery for injection of local anaesthetic.

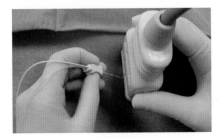

Fig. 8.24 The out-of-plane approach is more similar to the landmark techniques. A convenient location to perform the block is identified on ultrasound and the needle inserted from the medial side of the probe. Guiding the needle can be difficult because of the depth of the nerves from the skin. It can be difficult to manoeuvre the needle into a position so that the posterior nerves can be reached.

- Visualisation of the needle tip can be difficult because of the depth and angle of penetration and the probe may need to be angled back and forth to identify the tip of the needle.

The injection process

- Slowly inject local anaesthetic around the nerve cords by positioning the needle posterior and then superior to the axillary artery. Aspirate frequently to avoid inadvertent intravascular injection. If resistance to injection, severe paraesthesias or severe cramping pain are provoked in the limb during injection, immediately withdraw the needle by 1 to 2 mm to avoid intraneural injection.

- Observe the local anaesthetic spread during injection. A hypoechoic collection will appear adjacent to and then spread around the nerves.
- Observe the pattern of local anaesthetic spread around the target nerves during injection. Inject most of the local anaesthetic posterior to the subclavian artery.
- Reposition the needle at least once (from posterior to superior to the artery) to ensure complete circumferential local anaesthetic spread around the nerve roots. Local anaesthetic spread immediately posterior to the pectoral muscles or anterior to the axillary artery is commonly associated with block failure.

Axillary block

Landmark method

An axillary block is an excellent choice for anaesthesia of the forearm and hand, and is easily performed without the use of a nerve stimulator. However, because the musculocutaneous nerve leaves the brachial plexus sheath proximal to the site of injection, blind axillary brachial plexus block often results in a lack of anaesthesia of the volar aspect of the forearm below the elbow onto the thenar eminence.

Preparation

- Position the patient supine with the head facing away from the side to be blocked.
- Abduct the arm at the shoulder to 90° and flex the elbow to 90° and rest it comfortably. Do not abduct the shoulder joint by more than 90° because it makes palpation of the axillary artery pulse difficult and increases the risk of damage to the nerves during needle movement.
- With a pen, mark the significant landmarks (Fig. 8.25):
  - The axillary artery. If the location of the artery is not immediately apparent, ask the patient to adduct the arm against resistance. This tenses the pectoralis and coracobrachialis muscles and the pulse of the axillary artery can be found in the groove between these muscles.
  - The coracobrachialis muscle.

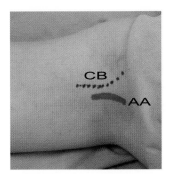

Fig. 8.25 The landmarks for the axillary block. The pulsation of the axillary artery (AA) and the muscle belly of coracobrachialis (CB) are marked on the skin.

Technique

- Prepare the field by cleaning the skin with an antiseptic solution and positioning sterile drapes.
- Identify the target area for needle insertion – just anterior to the pulsation of the axillary artery in the midaxillary fossa (the highest point of the axilla).
- Raise a superficial weal of local anaesthetic at the needle insertion site with a 27G needle.
- Press the axillary artery at the midaxillary fossa level with the index and middle fingers of the palpating hand and apply firm pressure. This shortens the distance between the skin and the brachial plexus and also stabilises the position of the artery during the needle advancement. This hand should not be moved during the block procedure, to allow for precise redirection of the needle if required.
- Puncture the skin at the target point (just anterior to the fingers of the palpating hand) with a 25 mm to 50 mm nerve-block needle. Advance the needle medially, slightly superiorly and slightly posteriorly at a 30° to 45° angle to the skin (Fig. 8.26A&B). The nerves will be found at a depth of 10–20 mm. The needle is advanced slowly until paraesthesias or appropriate muscle twitches are obtained or arterial puncture occurs.
- If the axillary artery is punctured before the plexus is encountered, then proceed with the transarterial technique: advance the needle through the axillary artery until blood can no longer be aspirated; inject one-third of the total volume of the local anaesthetic posterior and one-third anterior to the axillary artery on withdrawal of the needle.

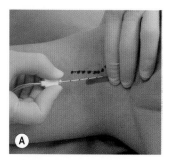

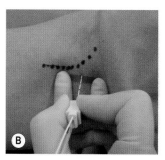

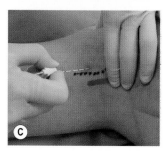

Fig. 8.26 The axillary block is performed with a puncture site immediately anterior to the axillary artery. The needle is either advanced medially at a 30° angle to the skin **(A)** or posterosuperiorly, perpendicularly to the skin **(B)**. The musculocutaneous nerve runs within the coracobrachialis muscle and can be blocked blindly or located with a nerve stimulator **(C)**.

- Aspirate. If no flashback of blood is obtained, inject 30 to 40 mL of local anaesthetic slowly with intermittent aspiration to rule out intravascular injection. Slow injection increases block success and decreases complications. If resistance to injection, severe paraesthesias or cramping pain sensations occur with initial injection, the needle should be withdrawn by 1 to 2 mm to avoid intraneural injection.
- The musculocutaneous nerve is often not blocked with the blind technique because it leaves the brachial plexus sheath proximal to the axilla. A block of the musculocutaneous nerve can be achieved with a separate injection by inserting the needle anterior to the artery into the substance of the coracobrachialis muscle (Fig. 8.26C). Twitches of the biceps indicate proximity to the nerve and 5 mL of local anaesthetic can be injected. In the absence of a nerve stimulator, a fan-technique injection of 5 mL of local anaesthetic may produce a successful block.

Ultrasound technique

The axillary approach can be used to block the terminal branches of the brachial plexus (the median, ulnar and radial nerves). The musculocutaneous nerve, which often leaves the brachial plexus proximal to the axilla, is commonly missed by the axillary approach but is easily blocked under ultrasound guidance.

Preparation

- Position the patient supine with the head facing away from the side to be blocked.
- Abduct the arm at the shoulder to 90° and flex the elbow to 90° and rest it comfortably.
- Use a linear high-frequency probe (10 to 15 MHz is ideal) and select an appropriate pre-set application.
- Identify the area to begin the scan – the midaxillary fossa. Perform a preliminary non-sterile survey scan to identify the relevant anatomy and optimise the image by adjusting depth of field (20 to 30 mm), focus point, and gain. Position the probe in the longitudinal plane (at right angles to the limb axis) to visualise the brachial plexus and axillary artery in a cross-sectional view (Fig. 8.27). Nerves in this region are predominantly hyperechoic but with a mixed echogenicity (honeycomb appearance) (Fig. 8.28A&B). The median and ulnar nerves lie superficial to the axillary artery and the radial nerve lies deep to the artery. The musculocutaneous nerve lies within the coracobrachialis muscle or in the fascia between biceps and

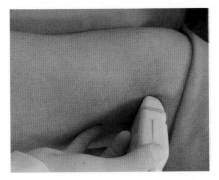

Fig. 8.27 The probe must be positioned as proximally as possible in the axilla in the longitudinal plane. The major landmark is the axillary artery, around which the nerves are arranged.

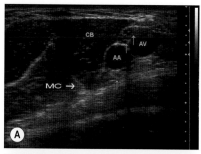

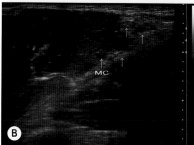

Fig. 8.28 The radial, ulnar and median nerves are located around the artery and need to be blocked individually. The position of the musculocutaneous nerve (MC) is variable within the coracobrachialis muscle (CB) and may be predominantly hyperechoic **(A)** or hypoechoic **(B)**.

coracobrachialis. Mark the best probe position on the skin with a pen, if required.

- Prepare the field by cleaning the skin with an antiseptic solution and positioning sterile drapes. Cover the probe with a sterile probe-sheath and apply sterile ultrasound gel to the area of the midaxillary fossa.

Technique

In-plane approach

- Identify the round or oval honeycomb nerves in their transverse axis in the axillary region and plan the approach: aim to block each nerve individually. Avoid excessive pressure on the probe as that will cause the axillary vein to collapse.
- Raise a weal of local anaesthetic at the needle insertion target with a 27G needle.
- Insert a 50 mm 22G nerve-block needle at the anterior end of the ultrasound probe (Fig. 8.29).

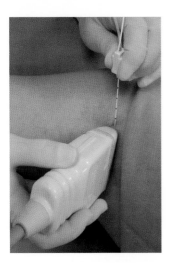

Fig. 8.29 The in-plane approach to the axillary block is performed from the anterior edge of the probe. The needle must be guided to each nerve (including the musculocutaneous nerve) so that they can be blocked individually.

- Advance the needle at a shallow angle because the nerves are very superficial in the axilla. The passage of the needle can be visualised in real time as it approaches the target nerves, while avoiding the axillary artery and vein.
- Manoeuvre the needle to the side of each nerve and aim to inject local anaesthetic around each nerve individually. Nerves can occupy a variable position in the axilla, but as long as each nerve is blocked, the procedure will be successful.
- Block the musculocutaneous nerve separately as it runs in the plane between the biceps and coracobrachialis muscles or within the substance of the coracobrachialis muscle.

Out-of-plane approach

- Identify the round or oval honeycomb nerves in their transverse axis in the axillary region and plan the approach: aim to block each nerve individually. Avoid excessive pressure on the probe as that will cause the axillary vein to collapse.
- Raise a weal of local anaesthetic at the needle insertion target with a 27G needle.
- Line up the target nerve in the centre of the screen and insert a 50 mm 22G nerve-block needle at the centre of the distal side of the ultrasound probe (Fig. 8.30).

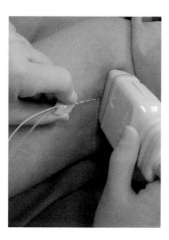

Fig. 8.30 The out-of-plane approach is performed from the distal side of the probe and is similar to the landmark technique. Again, each nerve needs to be blocked individually.

- Block each of the four nerves separately – this may require significant repositioning of the needle or a completely separate insertion point.
- Position the needle next to the nerve rather than head-on to it. It is easier to judge the needle position and has less risk of intraneural injection.

The injection process

- Slowly inject local anaesthetic around the nerve cords by positioning the needle adjacent to the nerve. Aspirate frequently to avoid inadvertent intravascular injection. If resistance to injection, severe paraesthesias or severe cramping pain are provoked in the limb during injection, then immediately withdraw the needle by 1 to 2 mm to avoid intraneural injection.
- Observe the local anaesthetic spread during injection. A hypoechoic collection will appear adjacent to and then spread around the nerves. If tissue expansion is not visible, this may represent an intravascular injection. Recheck the needle tip location relative to the axillary artery and vein before further injection.
- Inject 10 to 15 mL of local anaesthetic for each of the nerve locations.
- Reposition the needle at least once for each nerve to ensure complete circumferential local anaesthetic spread around the nerve.

Nerve blocks around the elbow

The nerves at the level of the elbow are shown in Fig. 8.31.

Landmark technique

The radial, median and ulnar nerves can be easily blocked just above or below the elbow. This will produce anaesthesia of the distal forearm, wrist and hand. These blocks can be used as 'rescue blocks' for

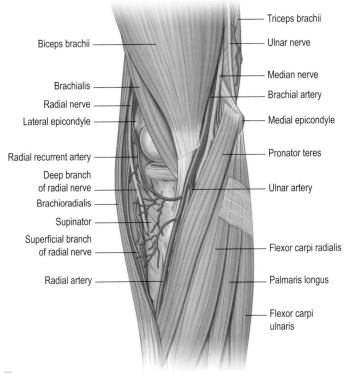

Biceps brachii

Brachialis
Radial nerve
Lateral epicondyle

Radial recurrent artery
Deep branch
of radial nerve
Brachioradialis
Supinator
Superficial branch
of radial nerve

Radial artery

Triceps brachii
Ulnar nerve

Median nerve
Brachial artery

Medial epicondyle

Pronator teres

Ulnar artery

Flexor carpi radialis

Palmaris longus

Flexor carpi
ulnaris

(A)

Fig. 8.31 Anatomical diagram of the nerves at the level of the elbow.

Continued

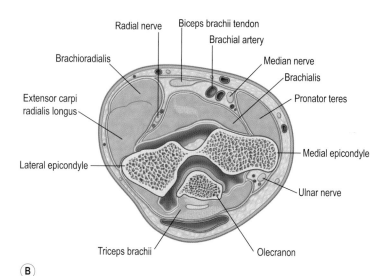

(B)

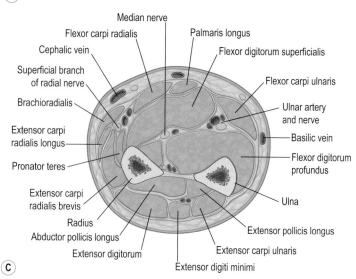

(C)

Fig. 8.31, cont'd. The cross-sectional anatomy of **(B)** the arm at the level of the forearm and **(C)** the forearm just distal to the elbow.

incomplete brachial plexus blocks, or used on their own for anaesthesia of the forearm and hand.

Preparation

- Position the patient supine or in semi-Fowler's position.
- Keep the forearm loosely at the patient's side or comfortably on a side-table. The elbow may need to be flexed and elevated above the patient's head for the ulnar nerve block.
- With a pen, mark the important landmarks:
  Ulnar nerve (Fig. 8.32):
  - The medial epicondyle of the humerus.
  - The medial edge of the olecranon.
  Median nerve (Fig. 8.33):
  - A line joining the medial and lateral epicondyles of the humerus, across the antecubital fossa.
  - The brachial artery pulsation 20 mm proximal to this line.
  Radial nerve (Fig. 8.34):
  - The lateral epicondyle.
  - The groove between the biceps tendon (medially) and the brachioradialis muscle (laterally) just above the level of the elbow joint (the biceps tendon can be accentuated by asking the patient to flex the elbow against resistance with the forearm supinated, and the brachioradialis with the forearm in 90° of pronation).

Technique

- Prepare the field by cleaning the skin with an antiseptic solution and positioning sterile drapes.

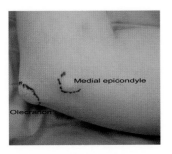

Fig. 8.32 The surface landmarks for the ulnar nerve at the elbow – the medial edge of the olecranon posteriorly and the medial epicondyle of the humerus anteriorly – form the boundaries of the ulnar groove through which the ulnar nerve runs.

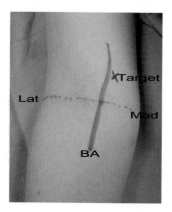

Fig. 8.33 The surface landmarks of the median nerve block at the elbow – just medial to the pulsation of the brachial artery (BA), 20 mm proximal to a line drawn between the lateral epicondyle (Lat) and medial epicondyle (Med) of the humerus.

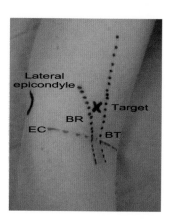

Fig. 8.34 The surface landmarks for the radial nerve block at the elbow include the lateral epicondyle of the humerus, the proximal elbow crease (EC), the muscle belly of brachioradialis (BR) and the biceps tendon (BT).

Ulnar nerve block at the elbow

- Position the patient's arm on the stretcher above their head, with the elbow flexed to 90°.
- Identify the target area for needle insertion – 10 to 20 mm proximal to the ulnar groove, **not** in the ulnar groove itself (there is a high risk of nerve penetration with the needle, as well as ischaemia from compartment syndrome) (Fig. 8.35A).
- Raise a superficial weal of local anaesthetic at the needle insertion site with a 27G needle.

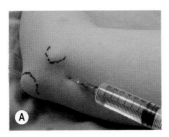
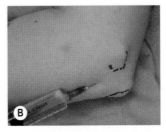

Fig. 8.35 The ulnar nerve may be blocked proximal **(A)** or distal **(B)** to the ulnar groove, but should not be blocked in the groove itself. The nerve lies very superficially in this region and blind injection into the region of the nerve has a high incidence of success.

- Advance the needle parallel to the long axis of the humerus through the subcutaneous tissue towards the ulnar groove. If paraesthesias or appropriate muscle twitches (in the hand) are produced then the position of the needle is confirmed.
- If the bone is contacted, withdraw the needle by 2 to 3 mm and proceed with the injection.
- Aspirate. If no flashback of blood is obtained, inject 3 to 5 mL of local anaesthetic slowly with intermittent aspiration to rule out intravascular injection. If blood is withdrawn, reposition the needle slightly and re-aspirate.
- Alternatively, the ulnar nerve may be blocked 10 to 20 mm distal to the ulnar groove, with the needle orientated either proximally or distally along the long axis of the forearm (Fig. 8.35B).

Median nerve block at the elbow

- Identify the target area for needle insertion – immediately medial to the pulsation of the brachial artery, 20 mm proximal to the intercondylar line (the proximal elbow crease) (Fig. 8.36).
- Raise a superficial weal of local anaesthetic at the needle insertion site with a 27G needle.
- Advance the needle posteriorly until the biceps fascia is punctured (5 to 10 mm depth).

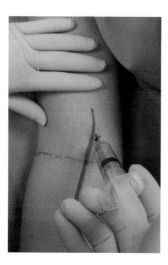

Fig. 8.36 The puncture site for the median nerve block at the level of the elbow is just medial to the brachial artery, 20 mm proximal to the elbow crease. The needle is advanced directly posteriorly through the fascia before injecting local anaesthetic.

- Aspirate. If no flashback of blood is obtained, inject 5 mL of local anaesthetic slowly with intermittent aspiration to rule out intravascular injection. If blood is aspirated, reposition the needle slightly and re-aspirate.
- Perform a block of the medial cutaneous nerve of the forearm at the same time. Withdraw the needle to the subcutaneous tissue and redirect it proximally in the subcutaneous plane between the head of the pronator teres muscle and the medial border of the biceps tendon. Aspirate. If no flashback of blood is obtained, inject 5 mL of local anaesthetic with a fan technique, slowly with intermittent aspiration to rule out intravascular injection.

Radial nerve block at the elbow

- Identify the target area for needle insertion – the groove between the biceps tendon and brachioradialis, 20 mm proximal to the flexor crease (the intercondylar line) (Fig. 8.37).
- Raise a superficial weal of local anaesthetic at the needle insertion site with a 27G needle.
- Puncture the skin and then advance the needle posteriorly and superiorly (proximally) towards the lateral aspect of the lateral epicondyle until bone is contacted (place a finger on the epicondyle and aim for that finger).

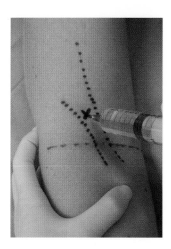

Fig. 8.37 The radial nerve is blocked at the elbow by inserting the needle in the groove between the biceps tendon (medially) and brachioradialis (laterally), 20 mm proximal to the elbow crease. It is directed posterolaterally towards a finger placed on the lateral epicondyle until the humerus is contacted. Local anaesthetic is injected close to the bone as the radial nerve runs against the humerus in this region.

- Withdraw the needle 1 mm, and aspirate. If no flashback of blood is obtained, inject 3 to 5 mL of local anaesthetic. Withdraw the needle slightly and redirect it 10 to 30 mm superiorly to contact the humerus again; pull back 5 mm and aspirate. If no flashback of blood is obtained, inject another 3 to 5 mL of local anaesthetic. If the aspiration is positive at any stage, reposition the needle slightly and re-aspirate before injecting.
- If a nerve stimulator is used, advance the needle until twitches causing dorsiflexion of the wrist are observed. Aspirate. If no flashback of blood is obtained, inject 5 to 10 mL of local anaesthetic.
- Perform a block of the lateral cutaneous nerve of the forearm at the same time as the radial nerve block at the elbow. Inject a fan of anaesthetic between the brachioradialis muscle and the lateral side of the biceps tendon.
- Also perform a block of the posterior cutaneous nerve of the forearm by injecting a weal of local anaesthetic solution subcutaneously from the lateral epicondyle to the olecranon.

Ultrasound techniques

The peripheral nerves of the brachial plexus at the level of the elbow are generally easy to visualise. They frequently have a heterogeneous echogenicity (honeycomb appearance) or are hyperechoic. They are also superficial (often within 10–20 mm from the skin surface) except in unusually muscular or obese patients.

If the nerve proves hard to locate, trace the course of the nerve by moving the probe proximally and distally. This is particularly relevant in the wrist or distal forearm where the nerves are surrounded by tendons. It may be possible to visualise the peripheral nerves in a long-axis view as well. Nerves in the forearm may exhibit a high degree of anisotropy and they may be hard to visualise on ultrasound unless the beam is at 90° to the nerve. If they are not easily visualised, it may be necessary to angle the probe proximally or distally in order to locate the nerves. Firm pressure applied by the ultrasound probe may also make the nerve stand out more prominently.

The easiest and most reliable method of performing the forearm block under ultrasound guidance is the mid-forearm ultrasound nerve block (FUN block). Performing the block procedure of the median and ulnar nerves at the level of the elbow is relatively straightforward, but the radial nerve procedure is more demanding and less successful. The radial nerve is more easily blocked in the mid-arm or the mid-forearm.

Ultrasound-guided blocks around the elbow

Preparation

- Position the patient supine or in semi-Fowler's position.
- Keep the forearm loosely at the patient's side or comfortably on a side-table. The elbow may need to be flexed and elevated above the patient's head for the ulnar nerve block.
- Use a linear high-frequency probe (10 to 15 MHz is ideal) and select an appropriate pre-set application.
- Identify the area to begin the scan for each nerve. Perform a preliminary non-sterile survey scan to identify the relevant anatomy and optimise the image by adjusting depth of field (20 to 30 mm), focus point, and gain. Position the probe in the longitudinal plane (at right angles to the limb axis) to visualise each nerve in a cross-sectional view. Nerves in this region are predominantly hyperechoic but with a mixed echogenicity (honeycomb appearance). Mark the best probe position on the skin with a pen, if required.
- Prepare the field by cleaning the skin with an antiseptic solution and positioning sterile drapes. Cover the probe with a sterile probe-sheath and apply sterile ultrasound gel to the area of the antecubital fossa.

Techniques

Ulnar nerve block at the elbow (Figs 8.38–8.41)

* Position the patient supine or in semi-Fowler's position and position the arm above the patient's head, with the elbow flexed at 90°.

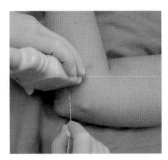

Fig. 8.38 The ulnar nerve can be blocked just below the elbow under ultrasound guidance with the probe held transverse to the limb axis. The out-of-plane technique is normally used, with the needle introduced from either the proximal or the distal side of the probe. The in-plane technique can also be used, with the needle advanced from the anterior edge of the probe. The nerve is easily visible in the ulnar groove as a round or oval structure with hyperechoic-predominant mixed echogenicity.

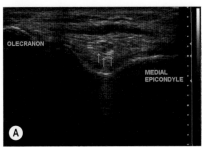

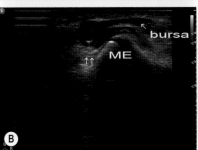

Fig. 8.39 The ulnar nerve just distal to the elbow, in the ulnar groove. **(A)** The ulnar nerve (arrows) between the olecranon and the medial epicondyle with their prominent acoustic shadows. **(B)** The medial epicondyle (ME) with an overlying fluid-filled bursa and the ulnar nerve in proximity. The olecranon is not visualised because of loss of contact between the probe and skin (because of a prominent olecranon in this case).

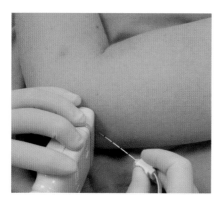

Fig. 8.40 The ulnar nerve may be blocked under ultrasound guidance at a point proximal to the elbow. Again, the out-of-plane approach is most commonly employed for this block, but either technique may be used. The needle is inserted from the proximal side (out-of-plane) or from the anterior edge (in-plane).

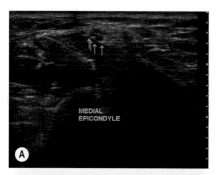

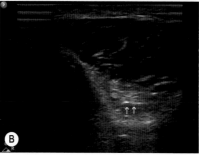

Fig. 8.41 The ulnar nerve is very superficial just proximal to the elbow **(A)** and deep to the triceps muscle slightly more proximally **(B)**. The arrows indicate the ulnar nerve, which is more hypoechoic in **(A)** and hyperechoic in **(B)**. The nerve can be traced proximally and distally to confirm its identity.

- Locate the ulnar nerve in the distal arm and proximal forearm (proximal or distal to the ulnar groove) with the ultrasound probe in the transverse plane to obtain a cross-sectional view of the ulnar nerve. It often has heterogeneous echogenicity at the level of the elbow. Align the nerve in the centre of the screen.
- Raise a weal of local anaesthetic subcutaneously at the target needle insertion site with a very fine needle (27G) on either the proximal or distal midpoint of the probe (the out-of-plane approach is more appropriate for this block, although the in-plane approach may be used).
- Advance the needle until it is in proximity to the nerve, aspirate, and then inject 3 to 5 mL of local anaesthetic slowly (with intermittent aspiration to rule out intravascular injection) while confirming that there is circumferential spread around the nerve. Insert the needle adjacent to the nerve rather than head-on and reposition the needle at least once in the injection process.
- If a nerve stimulator is used, look for twitches in the hand.

Median nerve block at the elbow (Figs 8.42A&B, 8.43A&B)

- Position the patient supine or in semi-Fowler's position and abduct the arm slightly and support it on the stretcher or a hand-table.
- Locate the median nerve in the distal arm and proximal forearm where it is superficial, heterogeneous in echogenicity, and lies immediately medial to the brachial artery.
- First locate the brachial artery (using colour Doppler if necessary), then identify the nerve medial to the artery.
- Scan proximally and distally to find a point where it is convenient to visualise and block the median nerve (normally just proximal to the elbow is most convenient). The median nerve can readily be traced from the axilla to the wrist. Align the nerve in the centre of the screen.
- Raise a weal of local anaesthetic subcutaneously at the target needle insertion site with a very fine needle (27G) on the distal midpoint of the probe (the out-of-plane approach is more appropriate for this block, although the in-plane approach may be used).
- Advance the needle until it is in proximity to the nerve, aspirate, and then inject 3 to 5 mL of local anaesthetic slowly (with intermittent aspiration to rule out intravascular injection) while confirming that there is circumferential spread around the nerve.

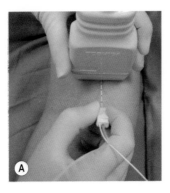 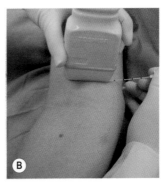

Fig. 8.42 The probe is positioned just proximal to the elbow crease in order to locate the brachial artery, which is the primary ultrasound landmark. Once the artery is identified, the median nerve can be located medial to the artery and either the out-of-plane **(A)** or in-plane **(B)** approach used to guide the needle adjacent to the nerve.

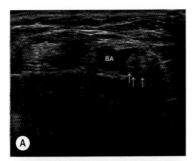

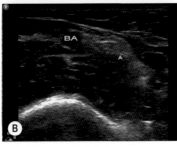

Fig. 8.43 The median nerve is usually immediately adjacent to the brachial artery (BA) **(A)** but may be separated medially in some patients **(B)** – the median nerve is 8 mm medial to the artery. The variability in echodensity of the nerves in different patients can be clearly seen here.

Insert the needle adjacent to the nerve rather than head-on and reposition the needle at least once in the injection process.
- If a nerve stimulator is used, look for twitches causing flexion of the fingers.

Radial nerve block at the elbow (Figs 8.44–8.47)
- Position the patient supine or in semi-Fowler's position and abduct the arm slightly and support it on the stretcher or a hand-table.
- Locate the radial nerve in the distal arm and proximal forearm between the brachialis and brachioradialis muscles where it has already divided into smaller superficial and deep branches. When traced proximally the nerve is larger, becomes deeper and then posterior to the humerus.
- The radial nerve can be blocked just above or just below the elbow at a point where it is convenient to visualise the nerves and perform the procedure.
- Align the radial nerve branches in the centre of the screen.
- Raise a weal of local anaesthetic subcutaneously at the target needle insertion site with a very fine needle (27G) on the distal midpoint of the probe (the out-of-plane approach is more appropriate for this block, although the in-plane approach may be used).

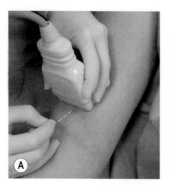 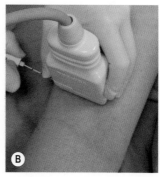

Fig. 8.44 The radial nerve can be blocked just above the elbow using the out-of-plane **(A)** or the in-plane **(B)** approach. The target can be seen between the muscle planes as two distinct nerves.

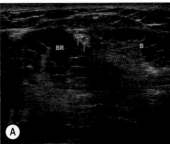

Fig. 8.45 **(A)&(B)** The ultrasound appearance of the structures surrounding the radial nerves varies greatly, depending on how proximal to the elbow the scan is performed. There are also considerable differences between patients, depending on gender and muscularity. The nerves consistently run in the fascial plane between brachioradialis (laterally) and brachialis (medially), however, and can readily be identified using these landmarks.

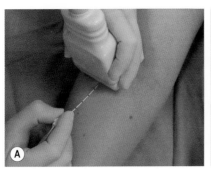

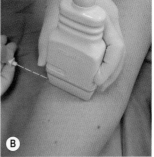

Fig. 8.46 The radial nerve can also be blocked just distal to the elbow using the out-of-plane **(A)** or the in-plane **(B)** approach. The nerves can be identified between the muscle planes in the same manner as just proximal to the elbow.

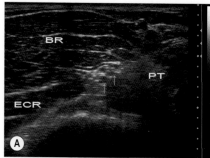

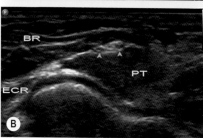

Fig. 8.47 (A)&(B) The location of the radial nerve immediately inferior to the elbow is very similar to that above the elbow, and the nerves can easily be traced proximally and distally to confirm their identity.
The nerves lie between brachioradialis (BR – superficial and lateral), extensor carpi radialis longus (ECR – deep and lateral) and pronator teres (PT – medially). The interface between these muscles forms a distinct ultrasound landmark.

- Advance the needle until it is in the same tissue plane as the nerves between the brachialis and brachioradialis muscles (above the elbow) or between brachioradialis and pronator teres (below the elbow). Aspirate and then inject 3 to 5 mL of local anaesthetic slowly (with intermittent aspiration to rule out intravascular injection) while confirming that there is tissue expansion within the correct plane and circumferential spread around the nerve. Insert the needle adjacent to the nerve rather than head-on and reposition the needle at least once in the injection process.
- If a nerve stimulator is used, look for twitches causing dorsiflexion of the hand.

Alternative radial nerve block in the mid-arm

The radial nerve can also easily be blocked in the distal third of the arm as it emerges from posterior to the humerus to run anterior to the lateral epicondyle between brachialis and brachioradialis.

Either internally rotate the arm and place the hand across the abdomen, or position the arm on the bed next to the patient with the elbow extended. Place the linear high-frequency transducer over the lateral aspect of the arm, about 100 mm proximal to the lateral epicondyle. The radial nerve can easily be identified as a hyperechoic oval structure lying close to the humerus posterior to the brachialis muscle and anterior to the triceps muscle. It can easily be blocked using either an in-plane or out-of-plane approach (Figs 8.48, 8.49A&B).

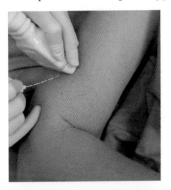

Fig. 8.48   The radial nerve is much easier to block in the mid-arm (mid-humeral block) than at the level of the elbow. The probe is placed on the lateral aspect of the arm, about 100 mm above the elbow, and the nerve located as it lies close to the humerus. The nerve is easily blocked using an in-plane or out-of-plane approach.

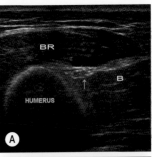

Fig. 8.49   (A)&(B) The radial nerve lies close to the humerus in the plane between brachioradialis (BR) and brachialis. It can consistently be located in this position. The position of the deep brachial artery should be evaluated using colour Doppler as it is often very close to the radial nerve. The nerve is most often hyperechoic at this level.

Forearm ultrasound nerve blocks (FUN block or mid-forearm block)

The radial, median, and ulnar nerves can reliably be blocked in the mid-forearm using ultrasound guidance. This produces anaesthesia of the hand, wrist and distal forearm (depending on how high the block is performed). This technique is somewhat easier than nerve blocks at the elbow and causes less discomfort to the patient than a wrist block.

Preparation
- Position the patient comfortably with their forearm by their side on the trolley or supported on a hand-table.
- Clean the entire forearm and apply sterile ultrasound gel from wrist to mid-forearm.
- Use a linear high-frequency probe with a sterile probe-cover for this block.

Techniques
Radial nerve FUN block (Figs 8.50, 8.51A&B)
- Locate the radial artery in the wrist, with the assistance of colour Doppler if necessary. It lies very superficially in this region, normally less than 10 mm deep.
- Trace the artery proximally into the mid-forearm (about 150 mm) and the radial nerve can be seen as a hyperechoic, honeycomb structure lying on the lateral (radial) aspect of the artery. It is usually immediately adjacent to the artery, but may also be situated slightly more laterally.
- Find a convenient position to perform the block.
- Block the nerve using either the out-of-plane or in-plane approach.
- Raise a weal of local anaesthetic subcutaneously at the target needle insertion site with a very fine needle (27G).
- Advance the needle until it is in proximity to the nerve, aspirate, and then inject 3 to 5 mL of local anaesthetic while confirming that there is circumferential spread around the nerve.

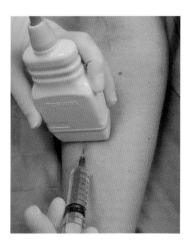

Fig. 8.50 The radial FUN block can be performed at any point in the forearm where the nerve is visualised clearly. Since the nerves are superficial, the out-of-plane approach is normally used (as illustrated here), but either approach can be used. The radial artery is the main ultrasound landmark for this block. It is identified in the wrist and traced proximally until the radial nerve is seen to appear on the lateral (radial) aspect of the artery.

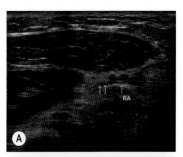

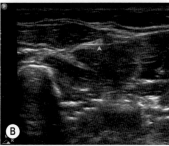

Fig. 8.51 The radial nerve (indicated by arrows in **(A)** and the arrowhead in **(B)**) is located on the radial (lateral) aspect of the radial artery (RA). The nerve is generally hyperechoic and may appear as an oval or round structure **(A)**, or a broader, flattened structure **(B)**.

Ulnar nerve FUN block (Figs 8.52, 8.53A&B)

- This block is the mirror-image of the radial nerve FUN block.
- Locate the ulnar artery in the wrist, with the assistance of colour Doppler if necessary. It lies very superficially in this region, normally less than 10 mm deep.
- Trace the artery proximally into the mid-forearm (about 150 mm) and the ulnar nerve can be seen as a hyperechoic, honeycomb structure lying on the medial (ulnar) aspect of the artery. It is usually immediately adjacent to the artery, but may also be as much as 10 mm more medially situated in the same tissue plane.
- Block the nerve using the out-of-plane approach.
- Raise a weal of local anaesthetic subcutaneously at the target needle insertion site with a very fine needle (27G).
- Advance the needle until it is in proximity to the nerve, aspirate, and then inject 3 to 5 mL of local anaesthetic while confirming that there is circumferential spread around the nerve.

Median nerve FUN block (Figs 8.54, 8.55A&B)

- Position the transducer transversely across the centre of the mid-forearm.
- The median nerve can be identified as an oval, hyperechoic structure lying between the muscle bellies of flexor digitorum superficialis (superficial), flexor pollicis longus (deep lateral) and

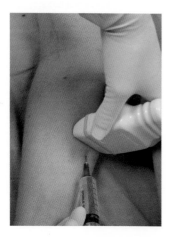

Fig. 8.52 The ulnar FUN block can also be performed at any level proximal to the mid-forearm. The ultrasound landmark for this block is the ulnar artery, which is often more medial than anticipated. This is identified in the wrist and traced proximally until the ulnar nerve is seen to appear on the ulnar (medial) side of the artery. The block can be performed using the out-of-plane technique (illustrated here) or the in-plane approach.

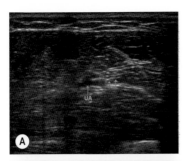

Fig. 8.53 The ulnar nerve (indicated by arrows in **(A)** and the arrowhead in **(B)**) is located on the ulnar (medial) aspect of the ulnar artery (UA), but may often not be immediately next to the artery, as is seen in these images. The nerve is generally hyperechoic.

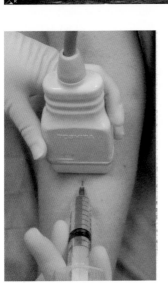

Fig. 8.54 The median FUN block, like the radial and ulnar blocks, can also be performed at any level proximal to the mid-forearm. There is no specific ultrasound landmark for this block but the median nerve can easily be identified as a hyperechoic round or oval structure within the muscles of the mid-forearm. The median nerve runs deeper than the radial and ulnar nerves. The probe is placed transversely in the centre of the forearm and angled proximally and distally until the nerve is identified. The block can be performed using the out-of-plane technique (illustrated here) or the in-plane approach.

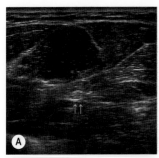

Fig. 8.55 The median nerve (indicated by arrows in (**A**) and the arrowhead in (**B**)) is located within the muscles of the mid-forearm. It is hyperechoic and usually easy to identify.

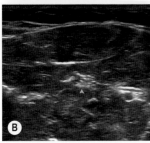

flexor digitorum profundus (deep medial) in the midline of the mid-forearm. It is deeper than the radial and ulnar nerves and is not associated with an adjacent vessel.

- Block the nerve using the out-of-plane approach.
- Raise a weal of local anaesthetic subcutaneously at the target needle insertion site with a very fine needle (27G).
- Advance the needle until it is in proximity to the nerve, aspirate, and then inject 3 to 5 mL of local anaesthetic while confirming that there is circumferential spread around the nerve.

Wrist block

The nerves at the level of the wrist are shown in Fig. 8.56.

Landmark technique

Regional blocks at the wrist are easy to perform with a blind landmark technique, do not require the use of a nerve stimulator, and are no

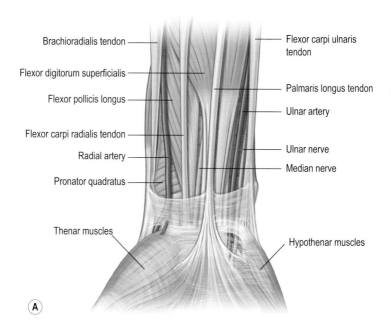

Brachioradialis tendon

Flexor digitorum superficialis

Flexor pollicis longus

Flexor carpi radialis tendon

Radial artery

Pronator quadratus

Thenar muscles

Flexor carpi ulnaris tendon

Palmaris longus tendon

Ulnar artery

Ulnar nerve

Median nerve

Hypothenar muscles

(A)

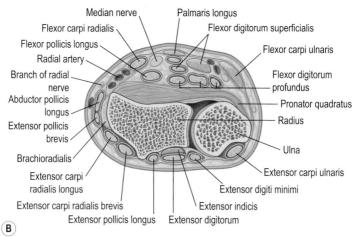

Median nerve

Flexor carpi radialis

Flexor pollicis longus

Radial artery

Branch of radial nerve

Abductor pollicis longus

Extensor pollicis brevis

Brachioradialis

Extensor carpi radialis longus

Extensor carpi radialis brevis

Extensor pollicis longus

Palmaris longus

Flexor digitorum superficialis

Flexor carpi ulnaris

Flexor digitorum profundus

Pronator quadratus

Radius

Ulna

Extensor carpi ulnaris

Extensor digiti minimi

Extensor indicis

Extensor digitorum

(B)

Fig. 8.56 Anatomical and cross-sectional diagram of the nerves at the level of the wrist.

simpler to perform with the assistance of ultrasound (tendons and nerves can be confusing at the level of the wrist)! It is important to be aware of potential compartment syndrome affecting the median and ulnar nerves.

The superficial branch of the radial nerve runs from the medial aspect of brachioradialis to pass between the tendon of the brachioradialis and radius to pierce the fascia on the dorsal aspect of the wrist. Just above the styloid process of the radius it gives digital branches to the dorsal skin of the thumb, index finger, and lateral half of the middle finger. Several of its branches pass superficially over the anatomic snuff box. The median nerve is located between the tendons of the palmaris longus and the flexor carpi radialis. The palmaris longus tendon is usually the more prominent of the two (although it may be absent in 10% of people) and the median nerve passes just lateral to it. The ulnar nerve passes between the ulnar artery and tendon of the flexor carpi ulnaris. The tendon of the flexor carpi ulnaris is superficial to the ulnar nerve.

A wrist block is useful for:

- rescue blocks for incomplete proximal blocks
- minor procedures (foreign body removal, laceration repair, fracture reduction) or dressings on the hand and fingers
- analgesia for injuries such as burns or more serious crushing injuries of the hand or fingers, until the patient can receive definitive surgery.

Preparation

- Position the patient supine with the arm positioned comfortably, slightly abducted and the wrist in slight extension (place a rolled-up towel under the wrist).
- Mark the important landmarks with a pen:
  - The radial styloid and the radial artery.
  - The tendons of palmaris longus and flexor carpi radialis. These can be accentuated by getting the patient to flex the wrist against resistance; or have the patient oppose the thumb and the little finger – this causes the tendon of palmaris longus to stand out.
  - The tendon of flexor carpi ulnaris and the ulnar artery. The flexor carpi ulnaris can be identified by asking the patient to flex the little finger at the metacarpophalangeal joint – the flexor carpi ulnaris becomes more prominent as it stabilises the pisiform bone during this manoeuvre.

Technique

- Prepare the field by cleaning the skin with an antiseptic solution and positioning sterile drapes.

Ulnar nerve block

- The ulnar nerve is anaesthetised by injecting local anaesthetic posteriorly and laterally to the tendon of the flexor carpi ulnaris muscle close to its distal attachment to the pisiform.
- The target point for needle insertion is either from the medial aspect of the wrist – the needle is inserted posterior to the tendon and advanced 5 to 10 mm to just past the tendon of the flexor carpi ulnaris – or, alternatively, the needle can be inserted on the volar aspect of the wrist just lateral to the tendon (between the tendon medially and the ulnar artery laterally) (Fig. 8.57A&B).
- Aspirate. If no flashback of blood is obtained, inject 3 to 5 mL of local anaesthetic slowly with intermittent aspiration to rule out intravascular injection.
- Inject 2 to 3 mL of local anaesthetic subcutaneously just superficial to the tendon of the flexor carpi ulnaris to block the cutaneous branches of the ulnar nerve which often innervate the hypothenar area.

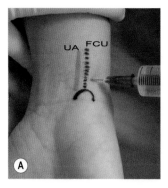 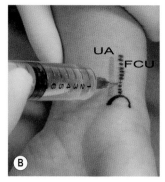

Fig. 8.57 The ulnar nerve lies just deep to the flexor carpi ulnaris (FCU) tendon and just medial to the ulnar artery (UA). It can be blocked from the medial **(A)** or anterior **(B)** aspect of the wrist with equal ease and success.

Median nerve block

- The target point for needle insertion is between the tendons of the palmaris longus medially and flexor carpi radialis laterally, on the volar aspect of the wrist, 20 to 30 mm proximal to the wrist crease (Fig. 8.58A&B).
- Advance the needle until it contacts the bone (usually at 5 to 15 mm depth), then withdraw the needle 2 to 3 mm.
- An alternative method is to advance the needle until the flexor retinaculum is penetrated with a 'pop'. The local anaesthetic can then be injected. Injections that are too superficial are less successful than those too deep as the retinaculum will prevent the local anaesthetic from penetrating to the nerve.
- Aspirate. If no flashback of blood is obtained, inject 3 to 5 mL of local anaesthetic slowly with intermittent aspiration to rule out intravascular injection.

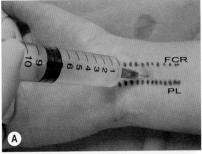

Fig. 8.58 The median nerve lies between the tendons of flexor carpi radialis (FCR) laterally and palmaris longus (PL) medially. The needle can be advanced from a more distal **(A)** or proximal **(B)** puncture site with equal success.

- Use a fan technique to increase the success rate of the median nerve block. Withdraw the needle to the subcutaneous tissue without removing it, redirect it 30° laterally, and advance again to contact the bone. After pulling back 1 to 2 mm off the bone, inject an additional 2 mL of local anaesthetic. Repeat the procedure with a medial redirection of the needle.

Radial nerve block

- This is essentially a field block and requires extensive subcutaneous infiltration because of the variable anatomic location of the distal radial nerve and its division into multiple, smaller, cutaneous branches (Fig. 8.59A&B).
- The target point for needle insertion is just proximal to the radial styloid (about 10 mm lateral to the radial artery).
- Inject 3 to 5 mL of local anaesthetic subcutaneously, aiming medially. Repeat the infiltration then aiming laterally, using an additional 3 to 5 mL of local anaesthetic.

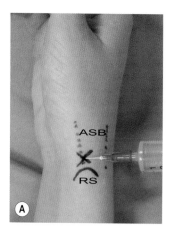

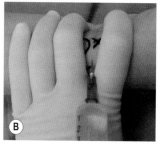

Fig. 8.59 **(A)** The radial nerve's superficial cutaneous branches can be blocked at the wrist by injecting a subcutaneous cuff of local anaesthetic at or just proximal to the radial styloid (RS). The cuff should be both anterior and posterior to the radial styloid. Avoid the dorsal branch of the radial artery in the anatomical snuff box (ASB). **(B)** An alternative method is to inject between two fingers that are used to apply firm pressure to the wrist. This forces the local anaesthetic to spread across the path of the cutaneous nerves in that region.

Metacarpal block

The fingers are supplied by the common digital nerves (derived from the ulnar and median nerves), which travel along the metacarpals to the metacarpophalangeal joint, where they divide into the volar and dorsal digital nerves.

A metacarpal block will provide complete anaesthesia to the digit, allowing for pain relief or procedures to be performed. There are three possible approaches:

- the palmar approach (painful)
- the dorsal webspace approach (less painful)
- the dorsal proximal approach (least painful).

Onset of anaesthesia occurs in 10 to 15 minutes; the duration of anaesthesia with lidocaine is 60 to 90 minutes and with bupivacaine is 3 to 6 hours. Do not use local anaesthetics that contain a vasoconstrictor – adrenaline (epinephrine) or noradrenaline (norepinephrine) – for fear of vascular spasm and necrosis of the fingertip. (This is not an evidence-based recommendation, but is common practice.)

Preparation

- Position the patient supine or in semi-Fowler's position with the arm slightly abducted. Support the forearm on an appropriate surface.
- Clean the entire hand with an appropriate antiseptic solution.

Technique

The palmar approach

- Insert the needle about 5 mm through the palmar skin just medial or lateral to the metacarpal neck (Fig. 8.60).
- Aspirate. If no flashback of blood is obtained, inject 1 to 2 mL of local anaesthetic slowly with intermittent aspiration to rule out intravascular injection.
- Repeat on the other side.

The dorsal webspace approach

- Hold the finger to be blocked with your thumb on the dorsal proximal phalanx and index finger on the volar aspect of the proximal phalanx.

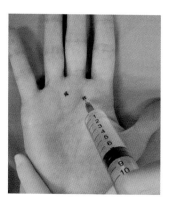

Fig. 8.60 This block is performed just distal to the distal palmar crease on each side of the metacarpal neck. The skin is penetrated to a depth of about 5 mm before injecting local anaesthetic.

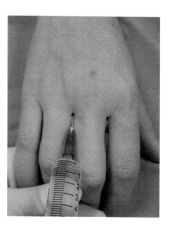

Fig. 8.61 This block is performed with a puncture site at the dorsal edge of the webspace on each side of the metacarpal of the finger to be blocked. The needle should be advanced close to the palmar skin surface before injecting local anaesthetic.

- Insert the needle on the medial or lateral aspect of the webspace, aiming towards the palmar skin – the needle should tent the skin, but not penetrate it (be careful of your finger!) (Fig. 8.61).
- Aspirate. If no flashback of blood is obtained, inject 1 to 2 mL of local anaesthetic slowly with intermittent aspiration to rule out intravascular injection.
- Repeat on the other side.

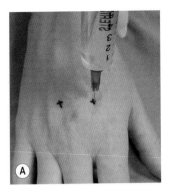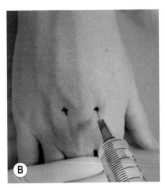

Fig. 8.62 The puncture site for injection is at the level of the metacarpal neck on each side of the ray to be blocked. The easiest approach for this block is to perform it with the patient's fingers pointing away, so that the needle can be angled slightly distally during advancement **(A)**. The injection from the distal side **(B)** is equally effective, however.

The dorsal proximal approach

- Position the patient's hand comfortable for the injection: stand either at the patient's side with the fingers pointing away, or facing the patient with the fingers pointed towards you.
- The target point for injection is approximately 25 mm proximal to the metacarpal head (Fig. 8.62A&B).
- Insert the needle at a slight angle distally until the deep fascia (the interosseus membrane) is penetrated (15 to 25 mm).
- Aspirate. If no flashback of blood is obtained, inject 2 to 4 mL of local anaesthetic slowly with intermittent aspiration to rule out intravascular injection.
- Repeat on the other side.
- This technique has less likelihood of causing raised compartment pressures in the hand because of the proximal injection site.

Digital nerve block (ring block)

A digital or ring block, as the name implies, is a technique of blocking the digital nerves in the finger or toe (where a ring would be) to achieve anaesthesia of the finger or toe. This technique is simple to perform and has very few complications. It is a commonly used and effective

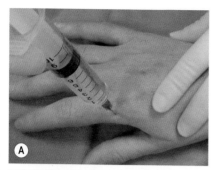

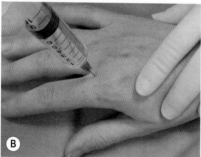

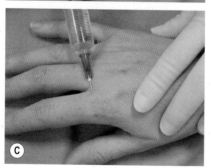

Fig. 8.63 The ring block is accomplished by depositing local anaesthetic around the base of the finger to block the palmar and dorsal digital nerves. Blocking the palmar nerves (**A,B**) will achieve anaesthesia of the anterior aspect of the finger aspect and the posterior aspect of the distal phalanx. To achieve anaesthesia on the posterior aspect of the proximal and middle phalanges, it is important to block the dorsal nerve network over the proximal phalanx (**C**).

method of anaesthesia employed in the ED for a wide variety of procedures on the digits. Several different techniques of digital block are described, and most are extremely effective.

Preparation

- Position the patient supine or in semi-Fowler's position.
- Abduct the arm slightly, pronate the hand and support it on a hand-table, or have it held by an assistant.

Technique (Fig. 8.63A–C)

- Clean the entire hand with a chlorhexidine in alcohol disinfectant solution.
- Insert a small (25G 35 mm) needle at a point on the dorsolateral aspect of the base of the proximal phalanx and raise a small skin weal of local anaesthetic.
- Advance the needle towards the phalanx until the bone is contacted; withdraw the needle 1 to 2 mm.
- Aspirate. If no flashback of blood is obtained, inject 1 mL of local anaesthetic slowly with intermittent aspiration to rule out intravascular injection.
- Inject an additional 1 mL of local anaesthetic as the needle is withdrawn.
- Repeat this procedure on the other side.
- A small weal of local anaesthetic over the dorsal aspect of the proximal phalanx may be needed to provide anaesthesia to the dorsal skin of the proximal and middle phalanges.
- Onset of local anaesthesia is from 5 to 20 minutes, depending on the type and volume of local anaesthetic used.

CHAPTER 9

Lower limb blocks

Landmark technique

A femoral nerve block is easy to master and has a very high success rate even in relatively inexperienced hands. It has a low risk of complications and has a significant clinical applicability in the ED for post-traumatic pain management of injuries of the femur, anterior thigh and knee. When a femoral nerve block is used in combination with a sciatic nerve block, anaesthesia of almost the entire lower limb distal to the mid-thigh can be achieved. The 3-in-1 block refers to the simultaneous blockade of the anterior branch of the obturator nerve, the lateral femoral cutaneous nerve and the femoral nerve with a single injection. This results from the medial and lateral spread of local anaesthetic injected around the femoral nerve.

The femoral nerve arises from the L2, L3 and L4 nerve roots. The nerve descends between the psoas and the iliacus muscles and passes deep to the inguinal ligament into the thigh (Fig. 9.1). At this point the femoral nerve is positioned immediately lateral to and slightly deeper than the femoral artery. The acronym **NAVY** is a useful reminder of the arrangement of structures from lateral to medial: **N**erve, **A**rtery, and **V**ein, with **Y** representing the midline.

A femoral block produces anaesthesia of the entire anterior thigh and most of the femur and knee joint, as well as to the skin on the medial aspect of the leg below the knee joint via the saphenous nerve.

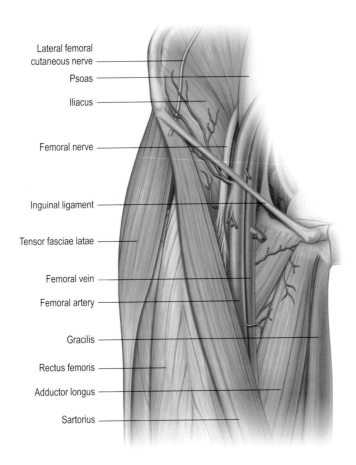

Lateral femoral
cutaneous nerve

Psoas

Iliacus

Femoral nerve

Inguinal ligament

Tensor fasciae latae

Femoral vein

Femoral artery

Gracilis

Rectus femoris

Adductor longus

Sartorius

Fig. 9.1 Anatomical diagram of the course of the femoral nerve in the proximal thigh.

Preparation

- Position the patient supine, with the hips and knees extended.
- Mark with a pen the important landmarks that are used
  to determine the target point for the needle insertion
  (Fig. 9.2):

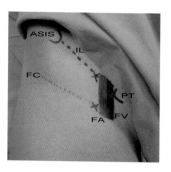

Fig. 9.2 The surface anatomy of the femoral nerve in the proximal thigh. The inguinal ligament (IL) extends from the anterior superior iliac spine (ASIS) to the pubic tubercle (PT), which lies just lateral to the pubic symphysis. The femoral nerve lies at the midpoint of this line just lateral to the femoral artery (FA) and femoral vein (FV). The target point for needle insertion may be at the level of the inguinal ligament (proximal cross) or at the level of the femoral crease (FC).

- The inguinal ligament – extending from the anterior superior iliac spine to the pubic tubercle.
- The femoral skin crease.
- The femoral artery pulsation at the femoral crease and inguinal ligament.
- The needle insertion point – immediately lateral to the femoral artery at the level of the inguinal ligament or femoral crease.

Technique

- Prepare the field by cleaning the skin with an antiseptic solution and positioning sterile drapes.
- Identify the target area for the initial needle insertion – a point immediately lateral to the arterial pulsation either at the level of the femoral crease or at the level of the inguinal ligament (Fig. 9.3A&B).
- Raise a superficial weal of local anaesthetic at the needle insertion site.
- Puncture the skin at the target point with a 25 mm to 50 mm nerve-block needle. Advance the needle posteriorly and slightly superiorly.
- If you are using a nerve stimulator, insert the needle using the same technique. Appropriate nerve stimulation must cause quadriceps contraction with movement of the patella. If the patella does not move, the sartorius muscle might have been stimulated.
- Aspirate. If no flashback of blood is obtained, inject 20 to 30 mL of local anaesthetic slowly with intermittent aspiration to rule out intravascular injection. Slow injection increases block success

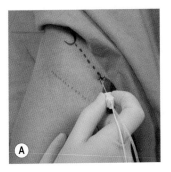 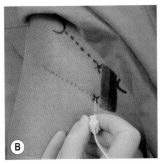

Fig. 9.3 The needle puncture site is just lateral to the femoral artery either at the level of the inguinal ligament or at the level of the femoral crease. The needle may be directed directly posteriorly **(A)** or posteriorly and superiorly **(B)**.

and decreases complications. If resistance to injection, severe paraesthesias or cramping pain sensations occur with initial injection, then the needle should be withdrawn by 1 to 2 mm to avoid intraneural injection. Use the higher end of the volume range if the 3-in-1 block is desired.

- Firm digital pressure applied distal to the injection site during injection and for several minutes thereafter increases the proximal, medial and lateral spread of local anaesthetic and increases the chances of achieving a 3-in-1 block.
- This block works well with smaller volumes of local anaesthetic, but larger volumes increase the likelihood of securing a block of the lateral femoral cutaneous nerve with resultant anaesthesia of the anterolateral aspect of the thigh.

Ultrasound technique

The use of ultrasound assistance for the femoral nerve block increases the success rate from 80% with the blind and nerve stimulator techniques to 95%. If ultrasound is used, then it is not necessary to use a nerve stimulator as well.

Preparation

- Position the patient supine with the hips and knees extended.
- Use a linear high-frequency probe (10 to 15 MHz is ideal) and select an appropriate pre-set application.

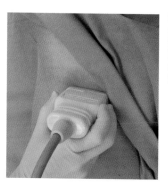

Fig. 9.4 The high-frequency linear probe is placed transversely on the anterior proximal thigh, at the level of either the inguinal ligament or the femoral crease. The initial ultrasound landmark to locate is the pulsatile femoral artery.

- Identify the area to begin the scan – the area between the inguinal ligament and the femoral crease.
- Perform a preliminary non-sterile survey scan to identify the relevant anatomy and optimise the image by adjusting depth of field (about 20 to 30 mm), focus point, and gain. Mark the best probe position on the skin with a pen, if required.
    - Place the probe transversely midway between the anterior superior iliac spine and the pubic tubercle (Fig. 9.4). Identify the pulsating femoral artery (lateral) and the compressible femoral vein (medially) with the assistance of colour Doppler if required (Fig. 9.5A–C). The femoral nerve is a triangular, often poorly defined, hyperechoic structure immediately lateral to the femoral artery. The femoral nerve may not be visibly distinct until the circumferential spread of local anaesthetic around the nerve. The position of the femoral nerve is generally easy to locate in this region.
    - The lateral femoral cutaneous nerve can often be identified during the survey scan: place the lateral edge of the probe against the anterior superior iliac spine just distal to the inguinal ligament. The nerve may be identified as a small hyperechoic structure between the fascia lata and the fascia iliaca, superficial to the sartorius muscle.
- Prepare the field by cleaning the skin with an antiseptic solution and positioning sterile drapes. Cover the probe with a sterile

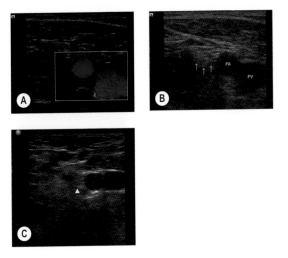

Fig. 9.5 The femoral artery and vein can be clearly seen and distinguished using colour Doppler **(A)**. The femoral vein (FV) lies closest to the midline, the femoral artery (FA) lateral to the vein, and the femoral nerve most lateral (arrows and arrowhead) **(B)** and **(C)**. The femoral nerve is not always clearly visible before the injection of local anaesthetic, but its position can be precisely inferred from the position of the femoral artery.

probe-sheath and apply sterile ultrasound gel to the area between the inguinal ligament and the femoral crease.

Technique

In-plane approach

- Identify the position of the femoral nerve in its transverse axis in an area convenient to block.
- Raise a weal of local anaesthetic at the needle insertion target with a 27G needle.
- Insert a 25 mm to 50 mm 22G nerve-block needle on the lateral end of the ultrasound probe.
- Advance the needle parallel to the probe towards the edge of the nerve while visualising the entire length of the needle in real time (Fig. 9.6).
- The lateral femoral cutaneous nerve may be blocked separately once the femoral nerve has been blocked.

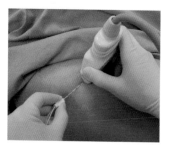

Fig. 9.6 To perform the in-plane approach, the needle is inserted from the lateral aspect of the probe and advanced under real-time guidance towards the lateral aspect of the nerve.

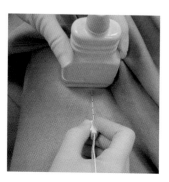

Fig. 9.7 The out-of-plane approach is performed from inferiorly and is very similar to the conventional technique. Aim for the lateral aspect of the femoral nerve. This is a very easy nerve block approach and is a good one for novices to attempt.

Out-of-plane approach

- Identify the position of the femoral nerve in its transverse axis in an area convenient to block.
- Line up the nerve target at the midpoint of the screen. The needle insertion point will correspond to the exact centre of the transducer.
- Raise a weal of local anaesthetic at the needle insertion target with a 27G needle.
- Insert a 25 mm to 50 mm 22G nerve-block needle on the inferior (distal) side of the ultrasound probe.
- Observe local tissue and needle movement as the needle is advanced towards the target. Aiming for the side of the nerve bundle rather than the centre makes needle placement more accurate (Fig. 9.7).
- Clear identification of the needle tip may require the probe to be angled back and forth.

- The femoral cutaneous nerve of the thigh may be blocked separately once the femoral nerve has been blocked.

The injection process

- Slowly inject local anaesthetic around the femoral nerve by positioning the needle adjacent to the nerve. Aspirate frequently to avoid inadvertent intravascular injection. If resistance to injection, severe paraesthesias or severe cramping pain are provoked in the limb during injection, then immediately withdraw the needle by 1 to 2 mm to avoid intraneural injection.
- Observe the local anaesthetic spread during injection. A hypoechoic collection will appear adjacent to and then spread around the nerve. Observe sheath distension and the formation of a hypoechoic ring of local anaesthetic solution around the hyperechoic nerve structures. Check to see if the local anaesthetic has spread around the lateral femoral cutaneous nerve – if not, it may need to be blocked separately.
- A lack of expansion of the tissue may indicate intravascular injection – aspirate and reposition the needle if necessary.
- Reposition the needle at least once to ensure complete circumferential local anaesthetic spread around the nerve roots.
- Scan proximally and distally to assess the extent of local anaesthetic spread.

Lateral femoral cutaneous nerve block

The lateral femoral cutaneous nerve arises from the L2 and L3 nerve roots and provides sensation to the lateral aspect of the thigh. It enters the thigh a variable distance medial to the anterior superior iliac spine (most commonly 10 to 15 mm, but as much as 50 mm) and deep to the inguinal ligament between the layers of the fascia lata and the fascia of the iliacus muscle. This block may be performed on its own or to complement a femoral nerve block.

Preparation

- Position the patient supine with the hips and knees extended.
- Mark with a pen the important landmarks that are used to determine the target point for the needle insertion (Figs 9.8, 9.9):
  - The anterior superior iliac spine.
  - The needle insertion point – 20 mm medial and 20 mm inferior (distal) to the anterior superior iliac spine.

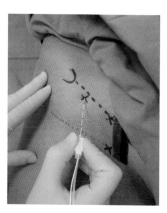

Fig. 9.8 The lateral femoral cutaneous nerve of the thigh may be blocked at a point 20 mm medial and 20 mm inferior to the anterior superior iliac spine. A fan-type of injection to disperse the local anaesthetic increases the chances of block success.

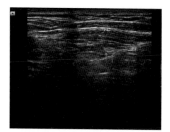

Fig. 9.9 The lateral femoral cutaneous nerve of the thigh can be visualised on ultrasound by positioning the probe immediately medial and inferior to the anterior superior iliac spine. The nerve can be seen between the fascia lata (FL) and the fascia iliaca (FI). It may be blocked using an in-plane or out-of-plane technique. If the nerve cannot be visualised, local anaesthetic can be deposited between the fascial layers about 15 to 20 mm medial to the anterior superior iliac spine.

Technique

- Prepare the field by cleaning the skin with an antiseptic solution and positioning sterile drapes.
- Identify the target area for the initial needle insertion – 20 mm medial and 20 mm inferior to the anterior superior iliac spine.

- Raise a superficial weal of local anaesthetic at the needle insertion site with a 27G needle.
- Puncture the skin at the target point with a 25 mm to 50 mm needle. Advance the needle posteriorly and slightly laterally until a 'pop' is felt as the nerve-block needle penetrates the fascia lata.
- Use a fan technique to inject 10 mL of local anaesthetic lateral and medial to the needle insertion point, both deep and superficial to the fascia lata. Aspirate intermittently to avoid intravascular injection.

Sciatic nerve block

Sciatic blockade (via the posterior, anterior or popliteal approach) has the potential to be one of the most commonly used regional anaesthetic techniques in the ED and can be invaluable for pain management following trauma to the lower limb (Fig. 9.10). This block is relatively easy and is associated with a high success rate when properly performed. It is particularly well suited for injuries to the leg, ankle, and foot. It provides complete anaesthesia of the leg below the knee with the exception of a medial strip of skin which is innervated by the saphenous nerve. When combined with a femoral nerve block or 3-in-1 block, anaesthesia of almost the entire lower limb distal to the mid-thigh is achieved. If spinal immobilisation procedures are required, rather use the anterior or the popliteal approach, which require less movement of the patient and the injured limb.

Posterior approach landmark technique

The traditional posterior approach to sciatic nerve blockade is relatively simple and successful but it has the disadvantage of requiring a significant repositioning of the patient, which might be difficult with an injured limb.

Preparation

- Position the patient in the lateral decubitus position with the side to be blocked uppermost. Flex the hip and knee to 90°.
- It is important that the patient remain in the same position once the landmarks have been marked. Small positional changes can result in a significant shift of the landmarks due to the movement of the skin, which can lead to difficulty in localising the sciatic nerve.
- Mark the important landmarks:
  - The greater trochanter.
  - The posterior superior iliac spine.

- The landmarks are easy to identify in most patients, but take care to palpate carefully when the landmarks are obscured in overweight or obese individuals.
  - Mark the innermost aspects of both landmarks. Marking the outer aspects will lead to inaccurate estimation of the position of the sciatic nerve.
  - Approach the greater trochanter from the posterior side when identifying and marking.

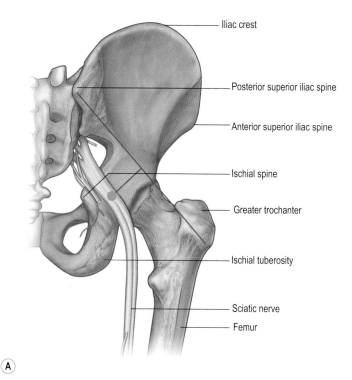

Iliac crest

Posterior superior iliac spine

Anterior superior iliac spine

Ischial spine

Greater trochanter

Ischial tuberosity

Sciatic nerve

Femur

(A)

Fig. 9.10 **(A)** Posterior view of the course of the sciatic nerve in the pelvis and proximal thigh. The red line indicates the landmarks for the posterior approach to this block.

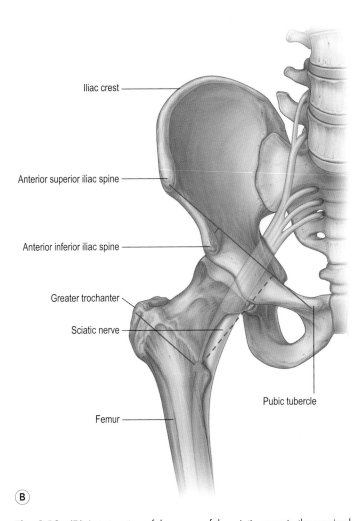

Iliac crest

Anterior superior iliac spine

Anterior inferior iliac spine

Greater trochanter

Sciatic nerve

Pubic tubercle

Femur

(B)

Fig. 9.10 **(B)** Anterior view of the course of the sciatic nerve in the proximal thigh. The landmarks used for the anterior approach to this block are indicated by the red lines. *Continued*

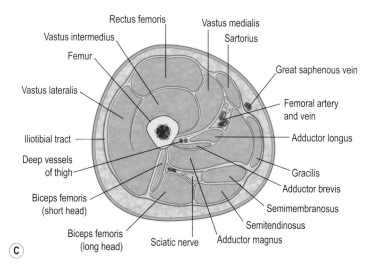

Fig. 9.10 (C) Cross-sectional anatomy of the proximal thigh.

- Approach the posterior superior iliac spine from the anterior side when identifying and marking.
- Draw a line from the greater trochanter to the posterior superior iliac spine; mark the midpoint of this line; the target point for needle insertion is 30 to 50 mm distal to this midpoint mark, perpendicular to the line (Fig. 9.11).

Technique

- Prepare the field by cleaning the skin with an antiseptic solution and positioning sterile drapes.
- Identify the target area for the initial needle insertion – a point 30 to 50 mm distal and perpendicular to the midpoint of a line joining the inner aspects of the greater trochanter and the posterior superior iliac spine.
- Raise a superficial weal of local anaesthetic at the needle insertion site with a 27G needle.
- Puncture the skin at the target point with a 75 mm to 100 mm nerve-block needle at a perpendicular angle to the spherical skin

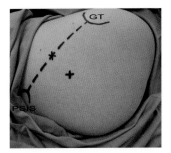

Fig. 9.11 With the patient in the lateral decubitus position, mark the midpoint of a line between the posterior aspect of the greater trochanter (GT) and the anterior aspect of the posterior superior iliac spine (PSIS). The target for needle puncture is a point 40 mm (30 to 50 mm) distal and perpendicular to this midpoint.

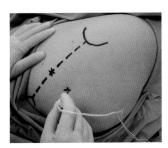

Fig. 9.12 The needle is inserted perpendicular to the skin and advanced directly in that plane until the sciatic nerve is encountered at a depth of 50 to 80 mm.

plane. Keep the needle at this angle while advancing it. The sciatic nerve should be encountered at 50 to 80 mm depth (Fig. 9.12).

- If you are using a nerve stimulator, use the same needle insertion technique and, once the target depth has been reached, look for twitches of the hamstrings, calf, foot, or toes. Gluteal twitches indicate that the needle is still too superficial. The use of nerve stimulation for the sciatic nerve can at times be misleading as the sciatic nerve is predominantly composed of sensory fibres. The needle may completely penetrate the nerve without producing muscle twitches!

- Aspirate. If no flashback of blood is obtained, inject 20 to 30 mL of local anaesthetic slowly with intermittent aspiration to rule out intravascular injection. Slow injection increases block success and decreases complications. If resistance to injection, severe paraesthesias or cramping pain sensations occur with initial injection, then the needle should be withdrawn by 1 to 2 mm to avoid intraneural injection.

- Onset of anaesthesia should occur in 15 to 30 minutes.

Posterior approach ultrasound technique

This block is one of the more difficult of the ultrasound-guided nerve blocks. Although the sciatic nerve is one of the largest peripheral nerves, it is often difficult to visualise because of the depth from the skin and because of the overlying adipose tissue.

Preparation

- Position the patient in the lateral decubitus position with the hip and knee flexed.
- Use a curvilinear probe (2 to 6 MHz) and select an appropriate pre-set application.
- Identify the area to begin the scan – the area between the ischial tuberosity and the greater trochanter (Fig. 9.13). The landmarks are easy to identify in most patients, but take care to visualise them carefully when excess adipose causes a poor image.
- Perform a preliminary non-sterile survey scan to identify the relevant anatomy and optimise the image by adjusting depth of field (about 40 to 80 mm), focus point, and gain. Mark the best probe position on the skin with a pen, if required.
  - Place the probe obliquely with the long axis parallel to a line between the ischial tuberosity and the greater trochanter in order to visualise the subgluteal space, which is an echolucent space deep to the gluteus maximus and superficial to the quadratus femoris muscles (Fig. 9.14A&B). The sciatic nerve, which is large, echogenic, wide and flat, always lies just medial to the midpoint of the echogenic fascia connecting the ischial tuberosity and the greater trochanter and appears as if it is protruding into the subgluteal space. There is an echogenic tendinous structure close to the greater trochanter

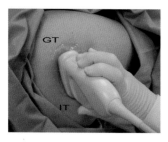

Fig. 9.13 The sciatic nerve is very deep when visualised with ultrasound from the posterior aspect and therefore a curvilinear low-frequency transducer is required. The probe is positioned transversely between the greater trochanter (GT) and the ischial tuberosity (IT) in order to visualise the sciatic nerve. The nerve is often very hard to locate and this block is difficult for novices.

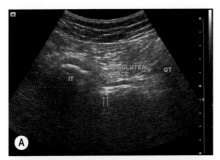

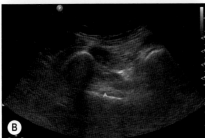

Fig. 9.14 (A)&(B) The sciatic nerve (usually) can be seen as a large hyperechoic oval structure in the medial half of the subgluteal space. The subgluteal space is an echolucent area between two 'tram-track' hyperechoic fascial planes running between the ischial tuberosity (IT) and the greater trochanter (GT). The arrows and arrowhead indicate the nerve.

that might be mistaken for the sciatic nerve but the sciatic nerve is always medial to the midpoint of the subgluteal space.

- Prepare the field by cleaning the skin with an antiseptic solution and positioning sterile drapes. Cover the probe with a sterile probe-sheath and apply sterile ultrasound gel to the area to be scanned.

Technique

In-plane approach

- Identify the position of the sciatic nerve in its transverse axis in an area convenient to block between the ischial tuberosity and the greater trochanter.
- Raise a weal of local anaesthetic at the needle insertion target point (the lateral edge of the probe) with a 27G needle.
- Insert a 75 mm to 100 mm 22G nerve-block needle on the lateral end of the ultrasound probe.

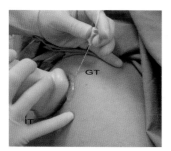

Fig. 9.15 The in-plane approach is most appropriate for this block as the needle has a long path to travel to the nerve. The needle is inserted at the lateral edge of the probe and guided in real time towards the edge of the nerve. The probe is held steadily between the greater trochanter (GT) and the ischial tuberosity (IT).

- Advance the needle parallel to the probe towards the edge of the nerve (rather than attempting to hit the nerve head-on) while visualising the entire length of the needle in real time (Fig. 9.15). Nerve movement may be noticed as the needle approaches the target.

Out-of-plane approach

- Identify the position of the sciatic nerve in its transverse axis in an area convenient to block between the ischial tuberosity and the greater trochanter.
- Line up the nerve target at the midpoint of the screen. The needle insertion point will correspond to the exact centre of the transducer.
- Raise a weal of local anaesthetic at the needle insertion target with a 27G needle.
- Insert a 75 mm to 100 mm 22G nerve-block needle on the inferior (distal) side of the ultrasound probe.
- Observe local tissue and needle movement as the needle is advanced towards the target. Aiming for the side of the nerve bundle rather than the centre makes needle placement more accurate.
- Clear identification of the needle tip may require the probe to be angled back and forth (Fig. 9.16).

The injection process

- Slowly inject local anaesthetic around the sciatic nerve by positioning the needle adjacent to the nerve. Aspirate frequently to avoid inadvertent intravascular injection. If resistance to

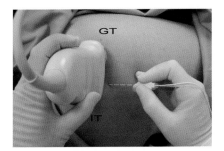

Fig. 9.16 The out-of-plane may be used and involves a shorter path from skin to nerve but the guidance of the needle requires movement or angling of the probe and inference of the needle-tip position from local tissue movement. The needle can be shaken slightly to accentuate tissue movement and aid in localisation of the tip. The needle is inserted from the distal side of the probe.

injection, severe paraesthesias or severe cramping pain are provoked in the limb during injection, then immediately withdraw the needle by 1 to 2 mm to avoid intraneural injection.

- Observe the local anaesthetic spread during injection. A hypoechoic collection will appear adjacent to and then spread around the nerve. Observe sheath distension and the formation of a hypoechoic ring of local anaesthetic solution around the hyperechoic nerve structures.
- Reposition the needle at least once to ensure complete circumferential local anaesthetic spread around the nerve roots.
- Scan proximally and distally to assess the extent of local anaesthetic spread. This is best achieved by rotating the probe by 90° to view the nerve in longitudinal section. Hypoechogenic local anaesthetic on both sides of the nerve will confirm correct placement and guarantee success of the block.

Anterior approach landmark technique

This approach has the advantage that it can be performed with the patient supine and does not require the repositioning of an injured limb.

Preparation

- Position the patient supine with the limb to be blocked in 45° of internal rotation if possible (this reduces the likelihood of needle contact with the lesser trochanter).
- Mark the important landmarks (Fig. 9.17):
  - The anterior superior iliac spine.
  - The pubic tubercle.
  - The greater trochanter.

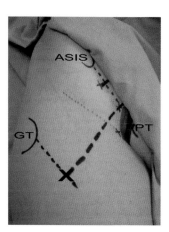

Fig. 9.17 The landmarks for the anterior sciatic nerve block should be marked with the lower limb maintained in 45° of internal rotation. A line between the anterior superior iliac spine (ASIS) and the pubic tubercle (PT) is divided into thirds. A perpendicular line dropped from the junction of the medial and middle thirds to intersect with a line from the centre of the greater trochanter (GT) marks the target point for needle insertion.

- Draw a line from the pubic tubercle to the anterior superior iliac spine; divide this line into thirds and drop a perpendicular line from the junction of the middle and medial thirds; draw a parallel line medially from the greater trochanter to intersect with the perpendicular. This marks the site of needle insertion.

Technique

- Prepare the field by cleaning the skin with an antiseptic solution and positioning sterile drapes.
- Identify the target area for the initial needle insertion – the junction of lines as described above.
- Raise a superficial weal of local anaesthetic at the needle insertion site with a 27G needle.
- Puncture the skin at the target point with a 75 mm to 100 mm nerve-block needle and advance the needle posteriorly and at a slight lateral angle.
- Advance the needle until contact is made with the femur. Retract the needle and redirect it medially until it deflects off the femur. Carefully advance the needle a further 5 to 10 mm (Fig. 9.18).
- The nerve stimulator should produce twitches of the calf, ankle or foot when the needle is positioned correctly.
- Aspirate. If no flashback of blood is obtained, inject 20 to 30 mL of local anaesthetic slowly with intermittent aspiration to rule out

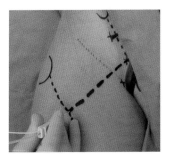

Fig. 9.18 The anterior sciatic nerve block is performed by advancing the needle directly posteriorly from the puncture site to contact the sciatic nerve just posterior to the femur. Internal rotation of the lower limb increases block success by decreasing the incidence of contact with the lesser trochanter of the femur.

intravascular injection. Slow injection increases block success and decreases complications. If resistance to injection, severe paraesthesias or cramping pain sensations occur with initial injection, the needle should be withdrawn by 1 to 2 mm to avoid intraneural injection.

- Onset of anaesthesia should occur in 15 to 30 minutes.

Anterior approach ultrasound technique

This technique is in some ways easier than the posterior ultrasound sciatic nerve block. It is performed with the patient supine without any repositioning necessary, the sciatic nerve is readily identifiable on ultrasound, and it may be performed from the same region as the femoral nerve block in the same sterile field (although a different probe needs to be used). The anterior approach to sciatic nerve blockade results in a lower incidence of blockade of the posterior cutaneous nerve of the thigh, however, and this should be considered when planning the block. The use of ultrasound for direct visualisation, and the medial needle insertion point (which avoids needle contact with the lesser trochanter), make this block much more successful than the landmark technique.

Preparation

- Position the patient supine. It may be necessary to abduct the opposite thigh to make space for the probe and to facilitate needle insertion and injection.
- Use a low-frequency curvilinear probe (2 to 6 MHz) as the nerve is often 80 to 100 mm below the skin and select an appropriate pre-set application.

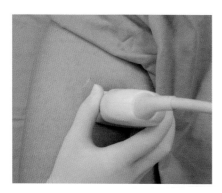

Fig. 9.19 The anterior sciatic nerve block is performed under guidance by a curvilinear low-frequency probe positioned transversely over the medial thigh as proximal as possible.

- Identify the area to begin the scan – position the transducer over the medial thigh as proximal as possible (Fig. 9.19).
- Perform a preliminary non-sterile survey scan to identify the relevant anatomy and optimise the image by adjusting depth of field (about 40 to 80 mm), focus point, and gain. Mark the best probe position on the skin with a pen, if required.
  - Locate and identify the femoral nerve and vessels – they look somewhat unfamiliar and much smaller when using the curvilinear probe. Use colour Doppler if necessary. This is important both in planning the path of the blocking needle as well as in locating the sciatic nerve.
  - Identify the femoral shaft as a bright hyperechoic crescent with a prominent acoustic shadow (Fig. 9.20A). This forms the lateral boundary of the area of interest.
  - Identify the sciatic nerve – it is a large, hyperechoic, oval structure that lies medial and deep to the femur (Fig. 9.20B). It lies in the tissue plane between the adductor muscles and hamstring muscles, which have a slightly different ultrasound appearance because of the direction of the muscle fibres.
  - If the sciatic nerve is difficult to locate at first, the right-angle method may prove helpful:
    - Visualise a line from the femoral neurovascular bundle to the centre of the shaft of the femur.
    - Visualise a medially-directed line originating from the centre of the femur at a right angle to the first line.
    - This line should run through the sciatic nerve within 50 mm of the femur.

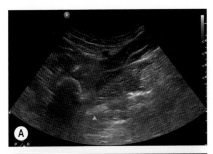

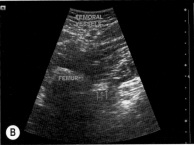

Fig. 9.20 (A)&(B) The initial landmark for this block is the acoustic shadow of the proximal femur, which is seen as a hyperechoic crescentic structure with a prominent acoustic shadow. The sciatic nerve is a large oval hyperechoic structure which is always medial and deep to the femur. It lies in a plane between two muscle groups which have a different echo-texture and is readily visualized.

- Prepare the field by cleaning the skin with an antiseptic solution and positioning sterile drapes. Cover the probe with a sterile probe-sheath and apply sterile ultrasound gel to the anteromedial thigh.

Technique

In-plane approach

The in-plane approach should be used for this block. Although the out-of-plane approach may be used, the depth of needle insertion makes this approach much more difficult.

- Identify the position of the sciatic nerve in its transverse axis in an area convenient to block in the proximal thigh. Plan the needle insertion point and path so that the femoral vessels and nerve are not pierced.
- Raise a weal of local anaesthetic at the needle insertion target point (the medial edge of the probe) with a 27G needle.

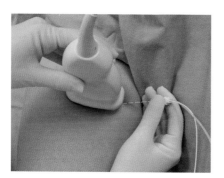

Fig. 9.21 The insertion site for this block is at the medial edge of the probe, well clear of the femoral vessels. The needle can be guided towards the medial edge of the nerve. A distinct 'pop' can be felt once the needle has penetrated the posterior fascia of adductor magnus to indicate proximity to the correct plane.

- Insert a 120 mm to 150 mm 22G nerve-block needle on the medial end of the ultrasound probe.
- Advance the needle parallel to the probe towards the edge of the sciatic nerve (rather than attempting to hit the nerve head-on) while visualising the entire length of the needle in real time (Fig. 9.21). Nerve movement may be noticed as the needle approaches the target.
- A distinct 'pop' should be felt as the needle penetrates each fascial layer, including the posterior fascia of adductor magnus which lies immediately anterior to the nerve.

The injection process

- Slowly inject 20 to 30 mL of local anaesthetic around the sciatic nerve by positioning the needle adjacent to the nerve. Aspirate frequently to avoid inadvertent intravascular injection. If resistance to injection, severe paraesthesias or severe cramping pain are provoked in the limb during injection, then immediately withdraw the needle by 1 to 2 mm to avoid intraneural injection.
- Observe the local anaesthetic spread during injection. A hypoechoic collection will appear adjacent to and then spread around the nerve. Observe sheath distension and the formation of a hypoechoic ring of local anaesthetic solution around the hyperechoic nerve structures.
- Reposition the needle at least once to ensure complete circumferential local anaesthetic spread around the nerve roots.
- Scan proximally and distally to assess the extent of local anaesthetic spread. This is best achieved by rotating the probe by

90° to view the nerve in longitudinal section. Hypoechogenic local anaesthetic on both sides of the nerve will confirm correct placement and guarantee success of the block.

Nerve blocks at knee level

There are three nerves that may be blocked at the level of the knee or the popliteal fossa: the saphenous nerve, the common fibular nerve (the common peroneal nerve) and the tibial nerve (Fig. 9.22). They may be

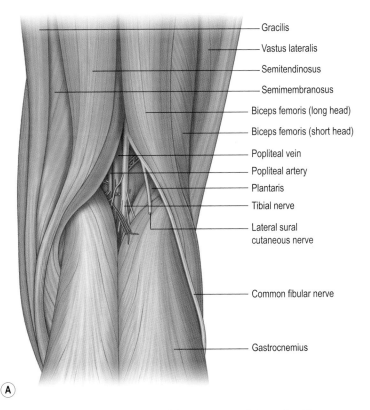

Gracilis

Vastus lateralis

Semitendinosus

Semimembranosus

Biceps femoris (long head)

Biceps femoris (short head)

Popliteal vein

Popliteal artery

Plantaris

Tibial nerve

Lateral sural cutaneous nerve

Common fibular nerve

Gastrocnemius

Ⓐ

Fig. 9.22 (A) Anatomical diagram of the nerves around the popliteal fossa.

Continued

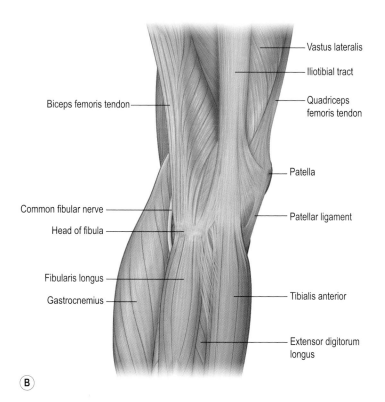

Fig. 9.22 **(B)** The path of the common fibular nerve on the lateral aspect of the knee.

blocked at the knee or alternatively the popliteal sciatic nerve may be blocked more proximally (the sciatic nerve branches into the common fibular nerve and the tibial nerve in the thigh, but they run together to the level of the knee). These nerve blocks will produce anaesthesia of the leg, ankle and foot.

Saphenous nerve block

This block should always be performed as distally as possible when done below the knee, as the saphenous nerve sends off numerous branches as soon as it becomes subcutaneous at the level of the knee.

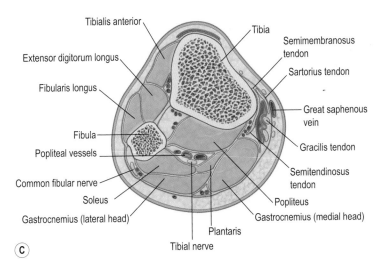

Fig. 9.22 (C) Cross-sectional anatomy of the proximal leg just distal to the knee.

It innervates the skin over the medial, anteromedial and posteromedial aspects of the leg, from the knee to the medial aspect of the hallux. In combination with a common fibular nerve and tibial nerve block this will produce anaesthesia of the leg, ankle and foot.

Preparation

- Position the patient supine on the trolley with the knee slightly flexed and elevated off the bed.
- Mark the important landmarks for this block (Fig. 9.23):
  - The tibial tuberosity.
  - The medial head of gastrocnemius.
  - The groove between sartorius and vastus medialis (for the above-knee approach).

Technique

- Prepare the field (the entire knee, proximal leg and distal thigh) by cleaning the skin with an antiseptic solution and positioning sterile drapes.

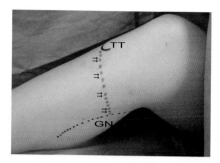

Fig. 9.23 The saphenous nerve block below the knee succeeds by blocking a neural network that is distributed between the tibial tuberosity (TT) and the medial head of gastrocnemius (GN). The arrows indicate the line of intended subcutaneous infiltration of local anaesthetic.

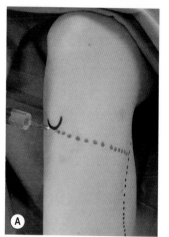

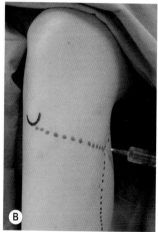

Fig. 9.24 (A)&(B) Local anaesthetic must be infiltrated subcutaneously along a line between the tibial tuberosity and the medial aspect of the calf. This may be done with several needle punctures or better with a longer needle such as a spinal needle that will require only a single puncture site.

- Identify the target point for needle insertion – just medial to the tibial tuberosity.
- Inject 5 to 10 mL of local anaesthetic as a deep subcutaneous line from the medial edge of the tibial tuberosity towards the posteromedial aspect of the calf (the medial head of gastrocnemius) (Fig. 9.24A&B). Inject slowly with intermittent aspiration to avoid inadvertent intravascular injection.

- An alternative technique is the paravenous approach (the saphenous nerve runs next to the saphenous vein at the level of the knee). Apply a tourniquet to the distal thigh to cause engorgement of the saphenous vein. Inject 3 to 5 mL of local anaesthetic around the vein on the medial aspect of the leg just distal to the patella. Aspirate frequently to prevent intravenous administration.
- A second alternative technique is to block the saphenous nerve above the knee in the groove between sartorius and vastus medialis. Position the patient supine with the knee extended. The groove, and the site for needle insertion, can best be identified 40 mm proximal to the superior aspect of the patella, and 40 mm medial to the midline. Insert the needle perpendicular to the skin to a depth of about 20 mm. Inject 5 to 10 mL of local anaesthetic using a fan technique, with frequent aspiration to prevent inadvertent intravascular injection.

Ultrasound technique

The saphenous nerve is readily blocked under ultrasound guidance even if the nerve itself cannot be visualised. This block is useful in the ED to provide anaesthesia for the management and repair of wounds over the anterior and medial aspect of the shin.

Preparation

- Position the patient supine with the limb slightly externally rotated.
- Use a linear high-frequency probe (10 to 15 MHz) and select an appropriate pre-set application.
- Identify the area to begin the scan – position the transducer over the anteromedial aspect of the distal thigh, about 50 mm proximal to the patella.
- Perform a preliminary non-sterile survey scan to identify the relevant anatomy and optimise the image by adjusting depth of field (about 20 to 30 mm), focus point, and gain. Mark the best probe position on the skin with a pen, if required.
  - Locate and identify the saphenous nerve in the groove between vastus medialis and sartorius (Figs 9.25, 9.26A&B). It is an oval, predominantly hyperechoic structure.
  - If the nerve cannot be visualised, local anaesthetic can be injected into the groove using a fan technique. An additional

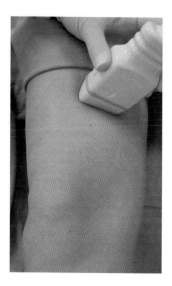

Fig. 9.25 The probe is positioned medially on the distal thigh. The initial ultrasound landmark is the vastus medialis muscle, which is followed medially to locate the groove between the vastus medialis and the sartorius muscle. The nerve can be found in this groove. This is a more advanced technique as the nerve may be difficult to visualise.

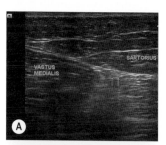

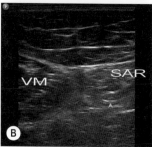

Fig. 9.26 **(A)&(B)** The groove between the vastus medialis (VM) and sartorius (SAR) muscles is easily identified, but the saphenous nerve might not be! It can often only be identified by tracing it proximally and distally to confirm it to be a contiguous neural structure.

5 to 10 mL of local anaesthetic injected posterior to sartorius increases the chance of block success.
- Prepare the field by cleaning the skin with an antiseptic solution and positioning sterile drapes. Cover the probe with a sterile probe-sheath and apply sterile ultrasound gel to the distal medial thigh.

Technique

Out-of-plane approach The out-of-plane approach is most convenient for this procedure (Fig. 9.27).

- Identify the groove between sartorius and vastus medialis and the saphenous nerve within the groove.
- Line up the nerve target at the midpoint of the screen. The needle insertion point will correspond to the exact centre of the transducer.
- Raise a weal of local anaesthetic at the needle insertion target with a 27G needle.
- Insert a 25 mm to 50 mm 22G nerve-block needle on the inferior (distal) side of the ultrasound probe.
- Observe local tissue and needle movement as the needle is advanced towards the target. Aim for the side of the nerve or the centre of the groove if the nerve is not visualised.

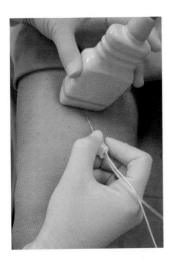

Fig. 9.27 The saphenous nerve is usually blocked with an out-of-plane-approach with the needle inserted from the distal side of the probe.

- Clear identification of the needle tip may require the probe to be angled back and forth.

The injection process
- Slowly inject 5 to 10 mL of local anaesthetic around the saphenous nerve by positioning the needle adjacent to the nerve. Aspirate frequently to avoid inadvertent intravascular injection. If resistance to injection, severe paraesthesias or severe cramping pain are provoked in the limb during injection, then immediately withdraw the needle by 1 to 2 mm to avoid intraneural injection.
- Observe the local anaesthetic spread during injection. A hypoechoic collection will appear adjacent to and then spread around the nerve. Observe distension within the groove and the formation of a hypoechoic ring of local anaesthetic.
- Reposition the needle at least once to ensure complete circumferential local anaesthetic spread around the nerve roots.

Alternative ultrasound technique (paravenous technique)
- Position a linear high-frequency 10–15 MHz transducer over the course of the saphenous vein in the proximal medial aspect of the leg, using sterile techniques.
- Optimise the scan image.
- Introduce a needle to each side of the saphenous nerve and inject 3 to 5 mL of local anaesthetic, with intermittent aspiration to avoid intravascular injection.

Common fibular nerve block

This nerve provides sensation to the lateral aspect of the leg, the dorsal aspect of the foot, and the first webspace. In combination with a tibial nerve and saphenous nerve block this will produce anaesthesia of the leg, ankle and foot.

Preparation

- Position the patient supine on the trolley with the knee slightly flexed and elevated off the bed.
- Mark the important landmarks for this block (Fig. 9.28):
  - The head of the fibula.
  - The biceps femoris tendon and insertion.

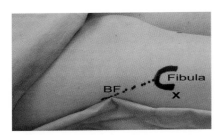

Fig. 9.28 The head of the fibula and the tendon of biceps femoris (BF) form the landmarks for this block. The knee may need to be flexed and extended to locate the exact positions of the landmarks. The 'X' marks the target site for needle insertion.

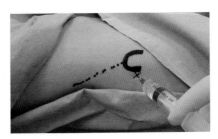

Fig. 9.29 The common fibular (peroneal) nerve block is performed by injecting local anaesthetic deep to the biceps femoris tendon where it attaches to the head of the fibula.

Technique

- Prepare the field (the entire knee, proximal leg and distal thigh) by cleaning the skin with an antiseptic solution and positioning sterile drapes.
- Identify the target point for needle insertion – immediately posterior to the head of the fibula, approximately 20 mm distal to the knee joint line.
- Insert the needle perpendicular to the skin and advance it approximately 10 mm, aiming under the tendon of biceps femoris (Fig. 9.29).
- If a nerve stimulator is used, look for twitches of the foot (dorsiflexion).
- Aspirate. If no flashback of blood is obtained, inject 5 to 10 mL of local anaesthetic slowly with intermittent aspiration to rule out intravascular injection. Slow injection increases block success and decreases complications. If resistance to injection, severe paraesthesias or cramping pain sensations occur with initial injection, then the needle should be withdrawn by 1 to 2 mm to avoid intraneural injection.

Tibial nerve block

The tibial nerve provides sensation to the sole of the foot. In combination with a common fibular nerve and saphenous nerve block this will produce anaesthesia of the leg, ankle and foot.

Preparation

- Position the patient prone on the trolley.
- Mark the important landmarks for this block (Fig. 9.30):
  - A line joining the medial and lateral condyles of the femur.
  - The midpoint of this line.
  - The pulsation of the popliteal artery.

Technique

- Prepare the field (the entire knee, proximal leg and distal thigh) by cleaning the skin with an antiseptic solution and positioning sterile drapes.
- Identify the target point for needle insertion – the midpoint of the line joining the femoral condyles and just lateral to the pulsation of the popliteal artery (Fig. 9.31).
- Advance the needle perpendicular to the skin to a depth of 15 to 30 mm in the average patient.
- If a nerve stimulator is used, look for twitches of the foot or toes.
- Aspirate. If no flashback of blood is obtained, inject 5 to 10 mL of local anaesthetic slowly with intermittent aspiration to rule out intravascular injection. Slow injection increases block success and decreases complications. If resistance to injection, severe paraesthesias or cramping pain sensations occur with initial

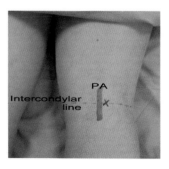

Fig. 9.30 The midpoint of a line joining the medial and lateral femoral condyles (the intercondylar line) marks the position of the tibial nerve and should be just lateral to the pulsation of the popliteal artery (PA).

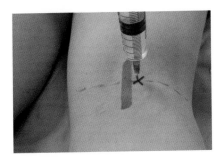

Fig. 9.31 The tibial nerve is blocked by advancing the needle directly anteriorly from a puncture site immediately lateral to the popliteal artery. The nerve is located 15 to 30 mm deep to the skin.

injection, then the needle should be withdrawn by 1 to 2 mm to avoid intraneural injection.

If an ultrasound is available, the popliteal sciatic block plus the saphenous block is a better option than attempting to block the tibial nerve at the level of the knee.

Popliteal sciatic nerve block

Since this procedure blocks the tibial nerve and the common fibular nerve as they run together in the thigh, it will produce anaesthesia of the entire foot, ankle and leg, with the exception of a strip of skin on the medial aspect of the leg. A saphenous nerve block will be required to complete the anaesthesia of the leg.

Landmark technique

Preparation

- Position the patient prone, with the feet hanging over the edge of the bed.
- Mark the important landmarks for this block (Fig. 9.32):
  - The proximal popliteal crease.
  - The tendons of semitendinosus and semimembranosus medially.
  - The tendon of biceps femoris laterally (these landmarks can be accentuated by asking the patient to flex the knee).
  - Draw a line parallel to the popliteal crease from the medial tendons to the lateral tendons, 70 mm proximal to the crease.
  - The midpoint of this line.

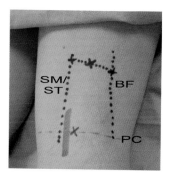

Fig. 9.32 The surface anatomy of the popliteal sciatic block: the needle entry point is at the midpoint of a line between the biceps femoris (BF) laterally and the semimembranosus (SM)/semitendinosus (ST) tendons medially, 70 mm proximal to the popliteal crease (PC).

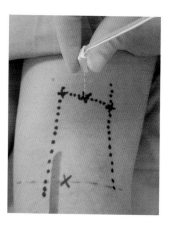

Fig. 9.33 The needle is advanced directly anteriorly until the sciatic nerve is located. If the femur is contacted without locating the nerve, the depth of penetration should be noted, as the nerve lies approximately halfway between the skin and the femur and the needle can be withdrawn to the correct plane.

Technique

- Prepare the field (the entire knee, proximal leg and thigh) by cleaning the skin with an antiseptic solution and positioning sterile drapes.
- Identify the target point for needle insertion – the midpoint of the line from medial to lateral tendons, 70 mm proximal to the popliteal crease.
- Advance the needle perpendicular to the skin to a depth of 20 to 40 mm in the average patient (Fig. 9.33).
- If a nerve stimulator is used, look for twitches of the foot or toes.

- Aspirate. If no flashback of blood is obtained, inject 5 to 10 mL of local anaesthetic slowly with intermittent aspiration to rule out intravascular injection. Slow injection increases block success and decreases complications. If resistance to injection, severe paraesthesias or cramping pain sensations occur with initial injection, then the needle should be withdrawn by 1 to 2 mm to avoid intraneural injection.

Ultrasound technique

The ultrasound-guided popliteal sciatic nerve block is a moderately difficult block as the popliteal sciatic nerve can be deceptively difficult to find for the novice ultrasonographer. It has the advantage that it can be performed in the prone patient and in the supine patient from the lateral side, or the medial side if required.

Preparation

- Position the patient prone with the feet hanging over the edge of the bed (or supine with the knee flexed to 90° and the foot flat on the bed for the supine approach).
- Use a linear high-frequency probe (10 to 15 MHz) and select an appropriate pre-set application.
- Identify the area to begin the scan – position the transducer over the posterior midline of the distal thigh, at least 70 mm proximal to the popliteal crease (Fig. 9.34A&B). The probe position is the same for both the prone and supine approaches.
- Perform a preliminary non-sterile survey scan to identify the relevant anatomy and optimise the image by adjusting depth of field (about 20 to 30 mm), focus point, and gain. Mark the best probe position on the skin with a pen, if required.
  - Locate and identify a transverse view of the sciatic nerve. Scan the sciatic nerve and take note of the point at which it divides into the tibial and fibular nerves (Fig. 9.35A&B). It is a round, hyperechoic structure that is lateral and superficial to the popliteal artery (which can be identified using colour Doppler if necessary). It is usually at a depth of about 30 mm from the skin, or about half the distance from the skin surface to the posterior cortex of the femur.
  - Aim to block the sciatic nerve before it divides. Scan proximally towards the apex of the popliteal triangle and follow the course of the nerve to determine an appropriate position for needle insertion.

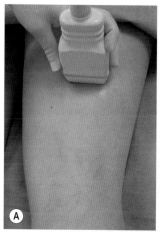
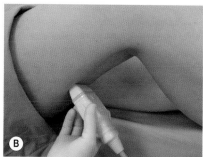

Fig. 9.34 The popliteal sciatic nerve may be blocked in the popliteal region with the patient prone (**A**), or supine with the knee flexed (**B**). The probe is positioned transversely in the mid to distal thigh midway between the biceps femoris and semimembranosus/semitendinosus tendons. The nerve has considerable anisotropy in this region and angling of the probe proximally and distally may be required to visualise the nerve.

- Prepare the field by cleaning the skin with an antiseptic solution and positioning sterile drapes. Cover the probe with a sterile probe-sheath and apply sterile ultrasound gel to the distal posterior thigh.

Technique

In-plane approach

This approach may be used with the patient prone and the knee extended or supine with the knee flexed and elevated off the bed.

- Identify the position of the sciatic nerve in its transverse axis in an area convenient to block, proximal to the division of the nerve (70 to 100 mm proximal to the popliteal crease).
- Raise a weal of local anaesthetic at the needle insertion target point (the lateral edge of the probe or a point away from the probe, more anterior on the lateral aspect of the thigh) with a 27G needle.

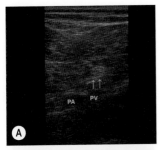

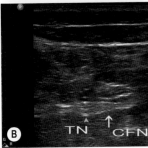

Fig. 9.35 The popliteal nerve is superficial and lateral to the popliteal artery **(A)**. The division of the sciatic nerve into the tibial nerve (TN) and common fibular nerve (CFN) can be seen in **(B)**.

- Insert a 50 mm to 75 mm 22G nerve-block needle on the lateral end of the ultrasound probe.
- Advance the needle parallel to the probe towards the edge of the nerve (rather than attempting to hit the nerve head-on) while visualising the entire length of the needle in real time (Fig. 9.36A&B). Nerve movement may be noticed as the needle approaches the target.

Out-of-plane approach

This approach can only be attempted with the patient in the prone position (Fig. 9.37).

- Identify the position of the sciatic nerve in its transverse axis in an area convenient to block, proximal to the division of the nerve (70 to 100 mm proximal to the popliteal crease).
- Line up the nerve target at the midpoint of the screen. The needle insertion point will correspond to the exact centre of the transducer.

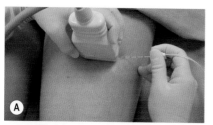

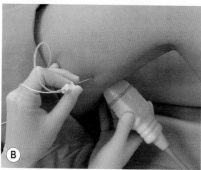

Fig. 9.36 The needle is advanced from the lateral side of the probe (prone position) **(A)** or from the lateral aspect of the thigh (supine position) **(B)** and guided under real-time visualisation to the lateral side of the nerve.

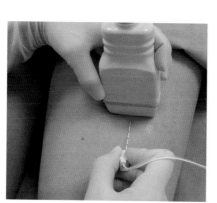

Fig. 9.37 The out-of-plane approach is performed from the distal side of the probe. This approach cannot be used for the supine patient.

- Raise a weal of local anaesthetic at the needle insertion target with a 27G needle.
- Insert a 50 mm to 75 mm 22G nerve-block needle on the inferior (distal) side of the ultrasound probe.
- Observe local tissue and needle movement as the needle is advanced towards the target. Aiming for the side of the nerve bundle rather than the centre makes needle placement more accurate.
- Clear identification of the needle tip may require the probe to be angled back and forth.

The injection process

- Slowly inject 20 to 40 mL of local anaesthetic around the sciatic nerve by positioning the needle adjacent to the nerve. Aspirate frequently to avoid inadvertent intravascular injection. If resistance to injection, severe paraesthesias or severe cramping pain are provoked in the limb during injection, then immediately withdraw the needle by 1 to 2 mm to avoid intraneural injection.
- Observe the local anaesthetic spread during injection. A hypoechoic collection will appear adjacent to and then spread around the nerve. Observe sheath distension and the formation of a hypoechoic ring of local anaesthetic solution around the hyperechoic nerve structures.
- Reposition the needle at least once to ensure complete circumferential local anaesthetic spread around the nerve roots.
- Scan proximally and distally to assess the extent of local anaesthetic spread. This is best achieved by rotating the probe by 90° to view the nerve in longitudinal section. Hypoechogenic local anaesthetic on both sides of the nerve will confirm correct placement and guarantee success of the block.

Ankle block

This block is straightforward to perform and produces anaesthesia of the superficial and deep structures of the foot distal to the ankle joint. It is highly successful using only the landmark technique, but is fairly uncomfortable for the patient because of the five injections required. The nerves that are blocked are the posterior tibial nerve, the deep fibular nerve (deep structures, bones, and cutaneous coverage of the sole and web between the first and second toes), and the superficial fibular, sural and saphenous nerves (cutaneous innervation of the foot) (Fig. 9.38). All superficial nerves of the foot are blocked by subcutaneous infiltration because they are no longer discrete nerves that can be blocked at the level of the ankle.

This is an important block for laceration repair to the sole of the foot because infiltration local anaesthesia is painful and ineffective.

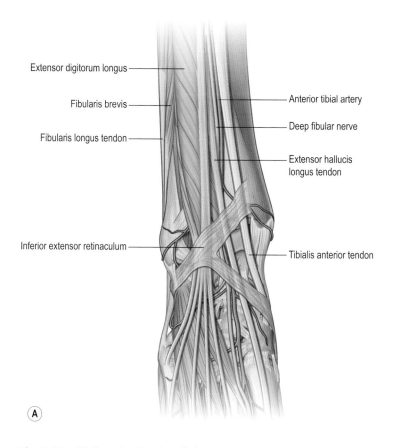

Extensor digitorum longus

Fibularis brevis

Fibularis longus tendon

Anterior tibial artery

Deep fibular nerve

Extensor hallucis longus tendon

Inferior extensor retinaculum

Tibialis anterior tendon

(A)

Fig. 9.38 (A) The path of the deep fibular nerve at the anterior aspect of the ankle.

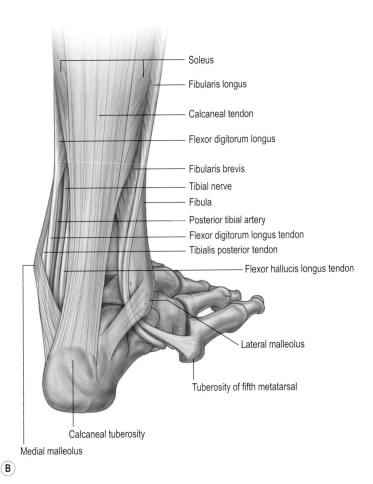

Soleus

Fibularis longus

Calcaneal tendon

Flexor digitorum longus

Fibularis brevis

Tibial nerve

Fibula

Posterior tibial artery

Flexor digitorum longus tendon

Tibialis posterior tendon

Flexor hallucis longus tendon

Lateral malleolus

Tuberosity of fifth metatarsal

Calcaneal tuberosity

Medial malleolus

(B)

Fig. 9.38 **(B)** The path of the tibial nerve on the posterior aspect of the ankle.
Continued

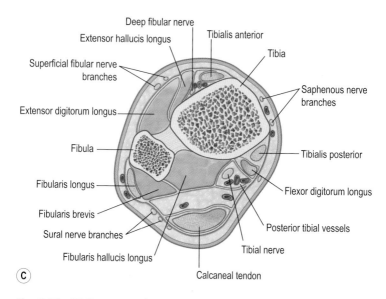

Deep fibular nerve
Extensor hallucis longus
Superficial fibular nerve branches
Extensor digitorum longus
Fibula
Fibularis longus
Fibularis brevis
Sural nerve branches
Fibularis hallucis longus

Tibialis anterior
Tibia
Saphenous nerve branches
Tibialis posterior
Flexor digitorum longus
Posterior tibial vessels
Tibial nerve
Calcaneal tendon

(C)

Fig. 9.38 **(C)** Cross-sectional anatomy of the distal leg just proximal to the ankle joint.

Deep fibular nerve block

Preparation

- Position the patient supine with the foot supported on pillows or rolled-up towels or with the knee flexed and the foot flat on the bed.
- Mark the important landmarks for this block (Fig. 9.39):
    - The tendon of extensor hallucis longus (EHL); do not confuse the tendon of tibialis anterior with that of EHL (EHL lies laterally to tibialis anterior).
    - The tendons of extensor digitorum longus (ask the patient to dorsiflex the toes but not the foot to identify these tendons).
    - The dorsalis pedis pulse.
    - The proximal ankle crease.
- Prepare the field (the foot, ankle and distal leg) by cleaning the skin with an antiseptic solution and positioning sterile drapes.

Technique

- Identify the target area for needle insertion – between extensor hallucis longus and extensor digitorum longus, immediately

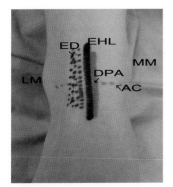

Fig. 9.39 The deep fibular nerve block is performed at the level of the proximal ankle crease (AC), which runs from the medial malleolus (MM) to the lateral malleolus (LM). The target point for needle puncture is just lateral to the pulsation of the dorsalis pedis artery (DPA), between the tendons of extensor hallucis longus (EHL) and extensor digitorum (ED).

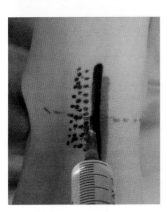

Fig. 9.40 The needle is advanced perpendicular to the skin immediately lateral to the dorsalis pedis artery. If the pulsation is not palpable (or if the artery is congenitally absent), the needle is inserted between the tendons of extensor hallucis longus and extensor digitorum.

lateral to the pulse of the dorsalis pedis artery at the level of the ankle crease in the anterior midline of the ankle.

- Raise a weal of local anaesthetic subcutaneously over the target area with a 27G needle.
- Insert a 22G needle in the groove just lateral to the extensor hallucis longus and advance until stopped by the bone (Fig. 9.40). Withdraw the needle 1 to 2 mm and inject 5 mL of local anaesthetic after aspirating to avoid intravascular injection.
- This block is a blind procedure, and a fan technique is recommended to increase the success rate. Withdraw the needle to the skin, redirect it 30° laterally and repeat the injection procedure. Repeat this with a medial redirection of the needle.

- Ultrasound technique: The fibular nerve is small at the level of the ankle, but can often be visualised in cross-section using ultrasound with a linear high-frequency probe positioned transversely across the ankle (Fig. 9.41). The nerve is to be found immediately lateral to the dorsalis pedis artery (Fig. 9.42A&B). It is hypoechoic at the level of the ankle. Block this nerve using the out-of-plane approach

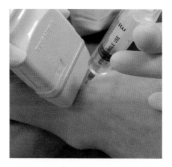

Fig. 9.41 To perform this block under ultrasound guidance, the probe is placed transversely over the ankle crease. The dorsalis pedis artery is located (using colour Doppler if necessary) and the nerve identified immediately lateral to the artery. The out-of-plane approach is used to inject local anaesthetic around the nerve.

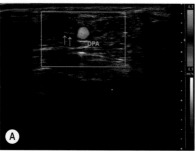

Fig. 9.42 The deep fibular nerve lies immediately lateral to the dorsalis pedis artery, superficial to the distal tibia. The arrows (**A**) and arrowhead (**B**) indicate the nerve. If the nerve cannot be seen, local anaesthetic can be injected around the dorsalis pedis artery.

by injecting 2 to 3 mL of local anaesthetic on each side of the nerve after aspirating to avoid intravascular injection. If the nerve cannot be identified, inject 2 to 3 mL of local anaesthetic on each side of the artery after aspirating to avoid intravascular injection.

Deep (posterior) tibial nerve block

Preparation

- Position the patient supine with the foot externally rotated and supported on pillows or rolled-up towels.
- Mark the important landmarks for this block (Fig. 9.43):
  - The medial malleolus.
  - The pulse of the posterior tibial artery.
- Prepare the field (the foot, ankle and distal leg) by cleaning the skin with an antiseptic solution and positioning sterile drapes.

Technique

- Identify the target point for needle insertion – the deep tibial nerve is located just posterior and distal to the medial malleolus, posterior to the pulse of the posterior tibial artery.
- Insert the needle in the groove posterior to the medial malleolus and advance it until contact with the bone. Withdraw the needle 1 to 2 mm and inject 5 mL of local anaesthetic after aspirating to avoid intravascular injection (Fig. 9.44).
- Use a fan technique to increase the success rate. Inject two additional boluses of 2 mL of local anaesthetic after anterior and posterior needle reinsertions, always after aspirating to avoid intravascular injection.

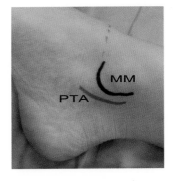

Fig. 9.43 The deep tibial nerve is located posterior to the posterior tibial artery (PTA) which runs posterior to the medial malleolus (MM).

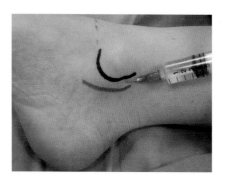

Fig. 9.44 Block the deep tibial nerve by injecting local anaesthetic anterior and posterior to the posterior tibial artery. The needle may be advanced perpendicularly to the skin until bone is contacted or advanced parallel to the artery into the same fascial plane before injecting.

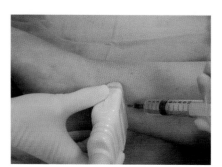

Fig. 9.45 The deep tibial nerve is visualised in cross-section immediately proximal to the medial malleolus. It lies posterior to the posterior tibial artery, which is easily identified using colour Doppler. Either the in-plane or more commonly the out-of-plane approach (illustrated here) can be used to guide the needle adjacent to the nerve.

- Ultrasound technique: Position a linear high-frequency probe transversely just proximal to the medial malleolus to visualise the tibial nerve in cross-section (Fig. 9.45). The nerve lies immediately posterior to the posterior tibial artery (Fig. 9.46A&B). Either the in-plane or out-of-plane technique can be used to guide the needle to the side of the nerve, where 5 mL of local anaesthetic can be injected after aspirating to avoid intravascular injection. Observe the spread of local anaesthetic around the nerve.

Superficial fibular, sural and saphenous nerve blocks

Blocks of the superficial fibular, sural and saphenous nerves, actually their distal superficial branches, are achieved using a simple circumferential injection of subcutaneous local anaesthetic (to all intents and purposes, a ring block around the ankle).

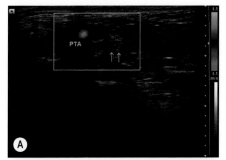

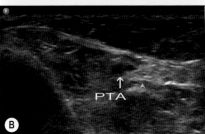

Fig. 9.46 The deep tibial nerve lies immediately posterior to the posterior tibial artery (PTA), posterior to the medial malleolus. **(A)** The arrows point to the nerve with the artery highlighted using colour Doppler. **(B)** The arrowhead indicates the nerve. If the nerve cannot be seen, local anaesthetic can be injected around the artery.

Preparation

- Position the patient supine with the foot supported on pillows or rolled-up towels – this will make access much easier.
- Make sure that you have access to both sides of the foot – bending over to block the other side can be very uncomfortable.
- Prepare the field (the foot, ankle and distal leg) by cleaning the skin with an antiseptic solution and positioning sterile drapes.

Technique

- *Superficial fibular nerve block* (Fig. 9.47): Insert the needle at the anterior tibial ridge and advance it laterally toward the lateral malleolus. Raise a subcutaneous weal during withdrawal of the needle with about 5 mL of local anaesthetic.
- *Saphenous nerve block* (Fig. 9.48): Insert a needle at the level of the medial malleolus and raise a ring of local anaesthetic from the point of needle entry to the Achilles tendon and then anteriorly to

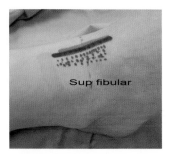

Fig. 9.47 The superficial fibular nerve can be blocked by a subcutaneous cuff of local anaesthetic on the anterolateral aspect of the ankle, as indicated by the yellow stripe.

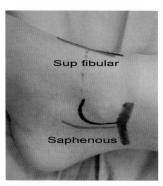

Fig. 9.48 The saphenous nerve is blocked with a subcutaneous cuff of local anaesthetic on the anteromedial aspect of the ankle, as indicated by the green stripe.

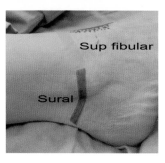

Fig. 9.49 The sural nerve is blocked with a subcutaneous cuff of local anaesthetic on the lateral aspect of the ankle, as indicated by the purple stripe.

the tibial ridge. Inject 5 mL of local anaesthetic during needle withdrawal.
- *Sural nerve block* (Fig. 9.49): Insert a needle at the level of the lateral malleolus and raise a weal of local anaesthetic posteriorly towards the Achilles tendon.

Metatarsal block

Anaesthesia of the toes can be achieved by means of a ring-block technique, in exactly the same way as for the fingers. A metatarsal block is an alternative that is less painful and more effective. This block may be performed with access through the webspace, or from the dorsal aspect of the foot, which is less painful.

Preparation

Position the patient supine, with the foot supported on a pillow or rolled-up towel – this will make for easier access.

Technique

- Clean the entire foot with a chlorhexidine in alcohol disinfectant solution.
- Identify the target points for needle insertion – immediately medial and lateral to the metatarsal of the digit to be anaesthetised, approximately two-thirds of the way from the base of the metatarsal to the head.
- Insert the needle close to the bone and advance it until near the plantar skin (tenting but not penetrating the skin) (Fig. 9.50).

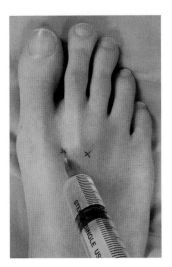

Fig. 9.50 The metatarsal block is performed on each side of the ray to be anaesthetised. The needle is advanced perpendicularly to the skin until the intermetatarsal interosseus membrane is punctured. Local anaesthetic is then injected to accomplish the block.

- Aspirate. If no flashback of blood is obtained, inject 3 to 5 mL of local anaesthetic slowly as the needle is slowly withdrawn towards the skin.
- Repeat this procedure on the opposite side of the metatarsal.

Digital nerve block (ring block) of the toes

A digital or ring block can be used to achieve anaesthesia of the toe. It is performed in much the same manner as a digital nerve block in the hand.

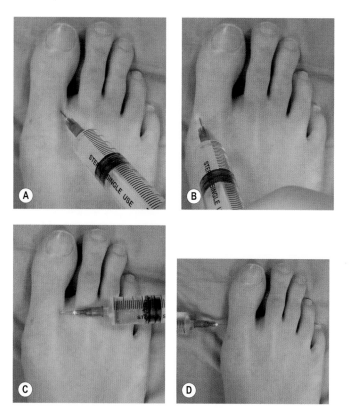

Fig. 9.51 **(A)–(D)** The digital (ring) block of the toe is used to inject a ring or cuff of local anaesthetic around the toe to provide distal anaesthesia.

Preparation

- Position the patient supine or in semi-Fowler's position.
- Position the foot comfortably in such a way that you have good access to the toes.

Technique (Fig. 9.51A–D)

- Clean the entire foot with a chlorhexidine in alcohol disinfectant solution.
- Insert a small (25G 35 mm) needle at a point on the dorsolateral aspect of the base of the proximal phalanx and raise a small skin weal of local anaesthetic.
- Advance the needle towards the plantar aspect of the toe.
- Aspirate. If no flashback of blood is obtained, inject 1 mL of local anaesthetic slowly with intermittent aspiration to rule out intravascular injection.
- Inject an additional 1 mL of local anaesthetic as the needle is withdrawn.
- Repeat this procedure on the other side.
- A small weal of local anaesthetic over the dorsal aspect of the proximal phalanx may be needed to provide anaesthesia to the dorsal skin of the proximal and middle phalanges.
- The hallux requires an additional weal of local anaesthetic on the plantar aspect of the toe.
- Onset of local anaesthesia is from 5 to 20 minutes, depending on the type and volume of local anaesthetic used.

CHAPTER 10

Miscellaneous blocks

Intercostal nerve block

This technique may be used to ease the pain of rib fractures, to allow the insertion of an intercostal drain or for other thoracic procedures. It can be a very easy procedure in relatively thin patients, but in patients with a muscular chest wall and obese patients it can be challenging with a high risk of pneumothorax. It should be avoided in patients with poor underlying respiratory function and those with coagulopathies.

Preparation
- Position the patient prone, in the lateral decubitus position (with the side to be blocked uppermost) or in a sitting position. Position the patient's arms in such a way as to pull the scapulae laterally.
- Mark the inferior margins of the ribs to be blocked just lateral to the paraspinal muscles (about 60 to 80 mm lateral to the midline for the inferior ribs and 40 to 70 mm for the superior ribs).
- The ribs can be counted from the 12th rib, or from the 7th rib, which is the most inferior rib covered by the inferior angle of the scapula.

Technique
- Prepare the field by cleaning the skin with an antiseptic solution and positioning sterile drapes.

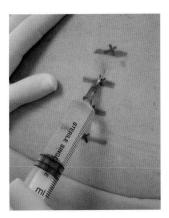

Fig. 10.1 Insert the needle at the top of the rib to be blocked. Carefully 'walk' the needle inferiorly until the inferior margin of the rib is passed. Maintain the superior angulation of the needle in order to place the needle close to the intercostal nerve.

- Identify the target points for needle insertion – the inferior margin of the rib, just lateral to the paraspinal muscles.
- Raise a weal of local anaesthetic at each anticipated needle insertion point with a 25G needle.
- Pull the skin about 10 mm superiorly and puncture the skin with the needle parallel to the sagittal plane.
- Angle the needle 20° to 30° superiorly. The needle may be grasped with an artery forceps or a needle holder for better control (be careful not to crush the needle).
- Advance the needle until the rib is contacted (about 10 mm in the average patient, more in muscular or obese patients).
- Release the retracted skin and 'walk' the needle inferiorly while maintaining the superior angulation of the needle (Fig. 10.1).
- Once the inferior edge of the rib has been reached, advance the needle about 3 mm – you might feel a 'pop' as the fascia is penetrated. The average distance from the posterior aspect of the rib to the pleura is 8 mm, so be careful not to advance the needle too far.
- Aspirate. If no flashback of blood is obtained, inject 3 to 5 mL of local anaesthetic slowly with intermittent aspiration to rule out intravascular injection.
- Repeat the procedure with the other ribs to be blocked and one rib above and one rib below these levels.

Miscellaneous blocks

- Local anaesthetic is rapidly absorbed after these blocks because of the high vascularity, so the toxic potential is high. Do not use more than 30 mL of bupivacaine for all the blocks combined.

Ultrasound technique

Preparation

- Position the patient prone, in the lateral decubitus position (with the side to be blocked uppermost) or in a sitting position.
- Position the patient's arms in such a way as to pull the scapulae laterally.
- Use a linear high-frequency probe (10 to 15 MHz is ideal) and select an appropriate pre-set application.
- Identify the area to begin the scan – the appropriate ribs to be blocked plus one rib above and one rib below.
- Perform a preliminary non-sterile survey scan to identify the relevant anatomy and optimise the image by adjusting depth of field (about 20 to 30 mm), focus point, and gain (Fig. 10.2). Mark the best probe position on the skin with a pen, if required.
  - Place the probe between the posterior axillary line and the paraspinal muscles in the longitudinal plane in a suitable position to obtain a transverse view of the rib to be blocked, the intercostal space and the rib below. Position the probe with the index marker superiorly so that the needle will be seen coming from right to left on the screen.

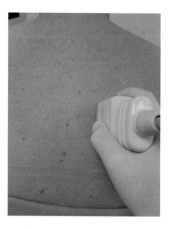

Fig. 10.2 Place the probe in the longitudinal plane over the region to be blocked. Optimise the image prior to sterile preparation.

- Prepare the field by cleaning the skin with an antiseptic solution and positioning sterile drapes. Cover the probe with a sterile probe-sheath and apply sterile ultrasound gel to the appropriate area.

Technique

This block should only be performed using the in-plane approach so that the movement of the needle can be visualised in real time in order to avoid accidental pleural puncture.

In-plane approach

- Identify the rib to be blocked in its transverse section, along with the rib below and the intercostal space in an area convenient to block.
- Ensure that the pleura is clearly visible (look for pleural sliding and comet tails).
- Identify the target point for needle insertion – the superior border of the rib inferior to the one to be blocked. Position the inferior edge of the probe at the superior edge of the rib below the one to be blocked (Fig. 10.3).
- Raise a weal of local anaesthetic at the needle insertion target with a 27G needle.
- Insert a 25 mm to 50 mm 22G nerve-block needle at the inferior end of the ultrasound probe.

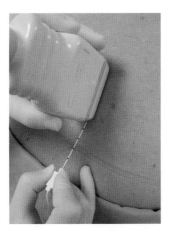

Fig. 10.3 Position the probe in the longitudinal plane in such a position that the needle can be inserted at the superior margin of the rib below. The path of the needle towards the intercostal groove can be visualised in real time and steered away from the pleura.

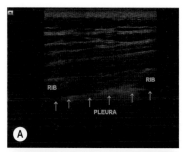

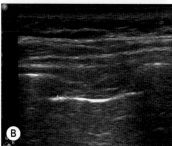

Fig. 10.4 **(A)&(B)** Transverse view of the posterior 5th and 6th ribs (the superior aspect is to the left of the image). The arrows point to the pleura – the movement of the visceral against the parietal pleura is clearly visible on real-time viewing. In **(B)**, the target point for injection, the intercostal groove, is indicated by the small arrowhead.

- Visualise the movement of the needle as it is advanced superiorly towards the intercostal groove (the nerve itself is not visible) (Fig. 10.4A&B). Ensure that the tip of the needle is visible at all times in order to avoid penetrating the pleura.
- Once the tip of the needle is in the costal groove, aspirate. If no flashback of blood is obtained, inject 3 to 5 mL of local anaesthetic slowly with intermittent aspiration to rule out intravascular injection.
- After the procedure is complete, confirm the absence of pneumothorax on the side of the procedure with standard ultrasound techniques.

Intrapleural block

An intrapleural block may be administered in two ways – through direct injection via a needle or catheter into the pleural space (which is rarely used in the ED) or through an intercostal drain (ICD) (thoracostomy tube) to relieve pain and discomfort from the ICD and from contused or fractured ribs. Rib pain and irritation of the parietal pleura from the ICD can cause significant symptoms, and delay re-expansion of a collapsed lung. This technique should not be used with a significant haemothorax if auto-transfusion may be considered, because of possible toxic side effects when the local anaesthetic is administered with the blood.

Technique

- Mix 10 mL of bupivacaine 0.5%, 10 mL of lidocaine 2% and 30 mL of normal saline. Ensure that these doses do not exceed the maximum dose for the patient's weight.
- Disconnect the intercostal drain from the bottle connection and inject the anaesthetic through the drain (during inspiration, to avoid it splashing in your face!).
- Clamp the ICD, reconnect the bottle and ask the patient to lie supine for 2 to 3 minutes, prone for 2 to 3 minutes and on each side for 2 to 3 minutes, then unclamp the drain.
- Unclamp the drain immediately at any stage if the patient becomes distressed.
- This block may be repeated after 12 hours if necessary.
- An alternative method is to insert a sealed butterfly needle through the ICD tube and tape it down. The local anaesthetic can be introduced through this needle without disconnecting the tube. Clamp the tube and reposition the patient as described above.

Penile block

This is a very useful technique to provide anaesthesia to the penis for circumcision, the dorsal slit procedure for paraphimosis, the management of priapism, laceration repair and for other penile trauma (entrapment in zippers, genital rings). There are several techniques described for the penile block and the two most common techniques are described below. The nerve block technique has the advantages of being less painful, easier to perform, and avoids the potential complications of penetrating the dorsal vessels of the penis with resultant haematoma. If adequate volumes are injected, both the dorsal and ventral nerves of the penis are blocked.

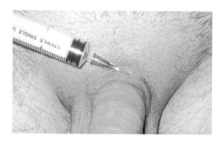

Fig. 10.5 Administer subcutaneous local anaesthetic on each side of the posterior midline at the base of the penis.

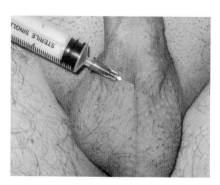

Fig. 10.6 Administer deep subcutaneous local anaesthetic on each side of the anterior midline of the penis.

The modified ring-block technique

- Position the patient supine – explain the procedure carefully!
- Clean the penis, scrotum and perineum with a chlorhexidine in alcohol solution.
- Raise three deep subcutaneous weals with about 2 mL of local anaesthetic solution (**without adrenaline** [epinephrine]): one on each side of the posterior midline at the base of the penis (Fig. 10.5) and one crossing the anterior median raphe at the junction of the penis and scrotum (Fig. 10.6).
- Join these weals with subcutaneous and intradermal rings of local anaesthesia.

Dorsal nerve of penis block

- Position the patient supine – explain the procedure carefully!
- Clean the penis, scrotum and perineum with a chlorhexidine in alcohol solution.

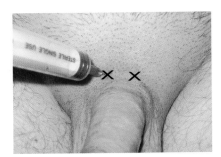

Fig. 10.7 Insert the needle on the posterior aspect of each side of the base of the penis as illustrated. The X marks the site of needle insertion on each side of the midline.

- Identify the target point for needle insertion – a point about 5 mm lateral to the midline at the level of the base of the penis (Fig. 10.7).
- Insert the needle perpendicular to the skin and advance it until the pubic symphysis is contacted. Withdraw the needle slightly and advance it approximately 5 mm, slightly laterally and inferiorly to the symphysis.
- Aspirate. If no flashback of blood is obtained, inject 5 to 8 mL of local anaesthetic slowly with intermittent aspiration to rule out intravascular injection.
- Repeat this technique on the opposite side.

Spermatic cord block

This block may be used to provide analgesia for injuries to the testes or to relieve the pain of the acute scrotum (after due consideration of the risks and benefits) to facilitate clinical examination.

Technique
- Position the patient supine – explain the procedure carefully!
- Clean the penis, scrotum and perineum with a chlorhexidine in alcohol solution.
- Identify the spermatic cord as it emerges from the external ring: grasp the cord and infiltrate 5 to 10 mL of local anaesthetic without adrenaline around the cord (Fig. 10.8). Aspirate frequently to exclude intravascular injection.
- Repeat on the opposite side if necessary.

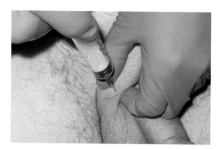

Fig. 10.8 Grasp the spermatic cord as proximal as possible and carefully inject local anaesthetic, while trying to avoid intravascular injection or injection into the vas deferens.

Intra-articular local anaesthesia

Injections of corticosteroids with local anaesthetic into the knee, ankle, shoulder or wrist have long been used for the treatment of inflammatory conditions. There is some suggestion that injection of local anaesthetic in the ED may benefit patients with painful injuries in these areas. There is as yet little published evidence about these techniques. There is good evidence, however, that the use of intra-articular local anaesthesia in anterior shoulder dislocation reductions is as good as conventional techniques of intravenous sedation and analgesia, but with a shorter stay in the ED as well as a lower cost.

Technique

- Sit the patient with their legs hanging over the side of the bed and their injured arm cradled in their lap. If this is not possible, let the patient lie on the uninjured side, facing away from you.
- Position yourself behind the patient.
- With a marking pen, mark the posterior aspect of the acromion as far as its lateral extension.
- Palpate the hollow area immediately inferior to the posterior edge of the acromion and mark the target area for needle insertion
  – 10 mm inferior to the acromion and 20 mm medial to the lateral edge (Fig. 10.9).
- Adhere to strict aseptic conditions: clean the area with chlorhexidine in alcohol, and use a gloved sterile technique.
- Insert the needle at the target area, aiming anteriorly and slightly inferiorly, under the acromion but superior to the head of the humerus. Insert the needle from 25 to 40 mm depending on the body habitus of the patient.

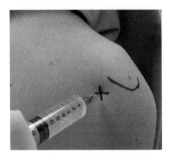

Fig. 10.9 The target point for injection is 10 mm inferior and 20 mm medial to the lateral end of the acromion. The needle is advanced anteriorly. In a patient with a dislocated shoulder, the subacromial space is exaggerated because of the subluxed humeral head.

- Aspirate. If there is no flashback of blood into the syringe, inject the local anaesthetic. There should be very low resistance to injection. If resistance is encountered, reposition the needle.
- Inject 20 mL of lidocaine 2% or 20 mL of bupivacaine 0.5% for a longer duration of analgesia.
- Onset of analgesia is from 10 to 30 minutes.

Haematoma block

This is a simple technique for producing anaesthesia to enable the reduction of a fracture. It may be used for many fractures but is most commonly used for distal radius fractures. It is safe and reliable both in adults and in children, with a low incidence of adverse events. Septic complications have not been commonplace following a haematoma block. It does not generate the density of anaesthesia as IVRA, but is much simpler and easier to use and gives enough analgesia for an adequate reduction in most cases.

Technique for distal radius haematoma block

- Use a sterile technique: clean the dorsal aspect of the distal forearm and wrist with an antiseptic solution. A sterile gloved technique should be used thereafter.
- Locate the fracture with gentle palpation, and correlate this with the findings from the lateral X-ray: it is often more proximal than expected.
- Identify the target area for needle insertion – the dorsal aspect of the radius 10 to 20 mm proximal to the fracture site.
- Raise a subcutaneous weal of local anaesthetic at the injection site.

- Puncture the skin with a 20G needle and advance it at a 45° angle towards the fracture.
- Angle the needle slightly more at the fracture site and advance it until an area of no resistance is encountered – the fracture haematoma.
- Aspirate – flashback of blood into the syringe confirms that the needle is in the haematoma.
- Use the intravenous lidocaine formulation for this block – introduction into the intraosseous space may cause systemic dissemination of the agent. The block is administrated by infiltrating 5 to 10 mL of lidocaine 1% (if this does not exceed the maximum permitted dose) directly into the fracture site. Analgesia occurs within 10 to 15 minutes after infiltration and will last for 30 to 60 minutes.
- If an ulnar styloid fracture is present, infiltrate 3 to 5 mL of lidocaine 1% into the fracture using the same sterile technique. This will further reduce the pain of reduction.

Ultrasound technique

Although the haematoma block is a fairly easy procedure to perform blind, ultrasound guidance can potentially increase the accuracy of needle placement. This will decrease the patient discomfort due to needle repositioning and decrease the incidence of failed blocks and therefore potential toxicity from repeated efforts. Ultrasound can also be used to evaluate the adequacy of the fracture reduction.

Ultrasound haematoma block for the distal radius

Preparation

- Position the patient supine.
- Rest the arm comfortably by the patient's side.
- Use a linear high-frequency probe (10 to 15 MHz is ideal) and select an appropriate pre-set application.
- Identify the area to begin the scan – the dorsal aspect of the distal radius over the fracture site.
- Perform a preliminary non-sterile survey scan to identify the relevant anatomy and optimise the image by adjusting depth of field (about 10 to 20 mm), focus point, and gain.
- Place the probe longitudinally over the distal radius to identify the cortical disruption and the adjacent hypoechoic haematoma.

- Prepare the field by cleaning the skin with an antiseptic solution and positioning sterile drapes. Cover the probe with a sterile probe-sheath and apply sterile ultrasound gel to the distal forearm.

Technique

In-plane approach
- Identify the fracture and adjacent haematoma.
- Identify the target site for needle insertion – 10 to 20 mm proximal to the fracture site. Position the proximal edge of the probe at the target site.
- Raise a weal of local anaesthetic at the needle insertion target with a 27G needle.
- Insert a 25 mm to 50 mm 22G nerve-block needle on the proximal end of the ultrasound probe.
- Advance the needle towards the haematoma while visualising the entire length of the needle in real time.
- Aspirate to confirm position within the haematoma, then inject 5 to 10 mL of lidocaine 1% into the haematoma.
- Confirm expansion of the hypoechoic haematoma during the injection of the local anaesthetic.

CHAPTER 11

Lara Goldstein

Procedural sedation and analgesia

Introduction

Pain is one of the most common reasons for patients to present to the ED and it is a reasonable expectation that their pain will be swiftly and skilfully managed. Similarly, patients in the ED often require diagnostic or therapeutic procedures that may cause apprehension or pain, or both. Patient dissatisfaction often relates to poor management of pain and anxiety or an inappropriate approach to the management of procedures. Emergency physicians are well qualified to administer procedural sedation and analgesia (PSA) while simultaneously monitoring the respiratory and cardiovascular status of both critically ill or injured patients and those with less dramatic but nonetheless painful conditions. Adequate analgesia and sedation for diagnostic and therapeutic interventions should be the standard of care in the ED.

The provision of safe and effective sedation and analgesia (for procedures or otherwise) is an important part of Emergency Medicine practice. The failure to adequately treat a patient's pain can have negative consequences, potentially affecting later psychological and physiologic responses and behaviours, especially in children. Appropriately treating pain and anxiety decreases patient suffering, facilitates medical interventions, increases patient/family satisfaction, improves patient care, and may improve patient outcome.

Providing effective and safe PSA in the ED is dependent on a number of factors:

- Appropriate patient selection and assessment.
- Appropriate selection and use of pharmacologic and non-pharmacologic agents.
- An appropriate environment for the procedure.
- Appropriate monitoring during and after the procedure.
- Appropriate post-procedure and pre-discharge evaluation.

There are many drugs and various non-pharmacologic modalities that can be used for PSA. The selection of a particular agent or modality is influenced by many factors, including patient characteristics (age, diagnosis, other illnesses, allergies) and the procedure to be performed (painful or painless, duration, depth of sedation required). Appropriate experience, staffing, equipment, monitoring and assessment are critical for safe and effective PSA.

Some of the myths that surround the use of analgesia in the ED negatively impact on the adequate and appropriate use of analgesic agents to treat pain and to be used as part of PSA. Some of these myths include:

- Children don't feel pain.
- Children don't remember pain.
- Patients can get addicted to opiates after a single dose.
- Opiates administered to patients can obscure the diagnosis of underlying pathology.
- PSA should be done only by anaesthetists.

What is PSA?

PSA involves the administration of sedative or dissociative agents with or without analgesic agents to induce a state that allows the patient to tolerate unpleasant or painful procedures. During the procedure, the patient maintains control of their airway and breathing because the protective airway and breathing reflexes are preserved. While PSA causes the patient to have a depressed level of consciousness, it allows them to maintain cardiorespiratory function.

Depth of sedation

Four levels of sedation have been defined by the American Society of Anesthesiologists (ASA):

- Minimal sedation (formerly anxiolysis). This is a state during which patients respond normally to verbal commands. Cognitive function and coordination may be impaired but ventilatory and cardiovascular functions are unaffected.
- Moderate sedation (formerly conscious sedation). This is a state of depressed consciousness during which patients respond purposefully to verbal or light tactile stimulation while maintaining protective airway reflexes. No cardiovascular or ventilatory assistance is required. In order to carry out potentially unpleasant procedures, moderate sedation is generally the goal.
- Deep sedation. This is a level of consciousness during which patients are not easily aroused and may need airway and/or ventilatory assistance. They may respond purposefully to repeated or painful stimulation. Cardiovascular function is usually maintained.
- General anaesthesia. This is a state of drug-induced loss of consciousness in which patients are not arousable and therefore require intervention for airway protection. They often have impaired cardiorespiratory function needing support.

These somewhat arbitrary categories are part of a continuum through which the patient may drift to a lighter or deeper sedative state. Individuals may also vary in their responses to the initial dose of a specific sedative with a resulting lighter or deeper sedation than intended. Physicians administering PSA should be proficient in the skills needed to rescue a patient at a level greater than the desired level of sedation. If moderate sedation is desired, the practitioner should be able to provide the skills needed to perform deep sedation. If deep sedation is required, the practitioner should be competent in the airway management and cardiovascular support involved in providing general anaesthesia.

Dissociative sedation, as produced by ketamine, is another form of sedation where a trance-like state is induced which provides analgesia and amnesia whilst leaving protective airway reflexes and cardiovascular stability unaffected. It cannot be categorised into any of the above levels of sedation.

How to perform PSA

The main aims for this chapter on PSA are to provide, or revise, some basic principles that can be used to improve patient care using an evidence-based approach. The physician should be able to ensure:

- Patient safety.
- Patient comfort.
- Physician comfort (i.e. decreased anxiety regarding the procedure and the patient's discomfort).
- An increased chance of successful completion of the intended procedure (although PSA does not necessarily guarantee that the procedure will not fail!).

In order to perform PSA safely in the ED according to evidence-based recommendations, there are seven key questions which need to be considered:

1. What are the human resources required to safely perform PSA in the ED?
2. How should patients be assessed *before* performing PSA?
3. Is fasting necessary before initiating PSA?
4. What equipment is required to perform PSA?
5. What monitoring is required to perform PSA in the ED?
6. How should respiratory status be assessed during PSA?
7. Can ketamine, midazolam, fentanyl, propofol and etomidate be safely administered to adults and children by emergency physicians in the ED?

So where do we start and how do we apply this in creating a plan for PSA? It's as easy as ABC (Fig. 11.1):

A – Assessment
B – Back-up/Background
C – Consent
D – Drugs
E – Equipment and monitoring
F – Fasting
G – Guidelines for discharge

Assessment

The assessment of the patient pre-PSA requires some additional information over and above the basic history and examination that has probably already been performed. Focus on the following:

- ASA physical status classification.
- Airway assessment.
- AMPLE history.

PROCEDURAL SEDATION PLAN CHECKLIST

NAME _____ AGE _____ WEIGHT _____ ✓

ASSESSMENT
    ASA Physical Status Classification
    Airway Assessment ☐
        Difficult Bag-Mask ventilation | B | O | O | T | S |
        Difficult intubation | M | M | A | P |
    AMPLE History
        Allergies _____
        Medication _____
        Past medical history _____
        Last Meal _____
        Events _____

BACK-UP Equipment?   Staff? ☐

CONSENT ☐

DRUGS
    SEDATION   ANALGESIA
    Etomidate |____| Fentanyl
    Propofol |____| (Morphine)
    Midazolam

    DISSOCIATIVE   OTHER _____
    Ketamine ☐   _____

EQUIPMENT & MONITORING
    PERSONNEL ☐   EQUIPMENT
                 Airway
    MONITORING   Drugs
    Pulse Oximetry   Resus
    Capnography   Anaphylaxis
                 Antidotes
              Defibrillator ☐

FASTING   Risk:Benefit considered? ☐

GUIDELINES FOR DISCHARGE
  1 Stable vital signs?
  2 Airway open and protected?
  3 Age-appropriate responses back to baseline?
  4 Adequate hydration?
  5 Supervised and/or able to understand discharge instructions?

Fig. 11.1 Procedural sedation plan checklist.

Children under the age of 2 years should generally receive PSA from a specialist with expertise in the management of infants.

ASA physical status classification

The ASA stratifies patients who will be undergoing anaesthesia according to a physical status classification (Table 11.1).

The limitation of this classification is that it was developed using general anaesthesia guidelines. Its utility in the emergent PSA application has not yet been formally established. Patients who fall into ASA class 3 or above have been shown to have a greater risk of sedation-related adverse events. It is generally accepted that patients in ASA classes 1 and 2 can safely undergo procedural sedation in the ED. ASA class 3 patients can be considered for ED procedural sedation – the potential risks and benefits should be taken into account, e.g. an awake patient with a supraventricular tachycardia requiring sedation for electrical cardioversion.

Airway assessment

In many ED scenarios the urgency of airway management does not always allow for the evaluation of a patient's airway in advance. This sometimes leads to the uncomfortable finding of an unanticipated difficult airway for which you are not prepared (unless you consider that *every* airway is going to be difficult!).

PSA can be considered to be semi-elective. It is therefore essential to assess your patient's airway prior to the performance of the procedure in order to have the relevant back-up equipment/medical staff available should the patient require airway and ventilatory management. This assessment should include predicting difficult bag–mask ventilation and intubation. Awareness of abnormal airway anatomy (e.g. micrognathia or macroglossia), the presence of dental appliances or

Table 11.1 ASA physical status classification	
Class 1	Normally healthy patient
Class 2	Mild systemic disease
Class 3	Severe systemic disease, but not incapacitating
Class 4	Severe systemic disease that is a constant threat to life
Class 5	Moribund, not expected to survive without the procedure

false teeth, a full beard, facial piercings, limited neck mobility, a short neck or history of stridor may all predict a difficult airway. The procedure should then be deferred to the operating theatre. The Mallampati score given for the view on mouth opening can also be added to the assessment process.

A useful aide-mémoire to recall the potential causes of difficult bag–mask ventilation is BOOTS.

Beard/Body piercings
Obesity
Old age (>65 years old)
Teeth abnormalities/Toothless
Snoring/Stridor/Syndromes

The mnemonic MMAP can be used to assess the patient's anatomy for possible difficult laryngoscopy.

Mallampati score. Class I and II generally correlate with easy direct laryngoscopy, while III and IV with difficult laryngoscopy.

Measurements **3-3-1.** Likely intubation difficulty can be envisaged if the patient can fit less than **3** of their own fingers in the hyomental area; less than **3** fingers between their upper and lower teeth (mouth opening); and has less than **1** cm of jaw protrusion (the ability to protrude the lower teeth anterior to the upper teeth).

Atlanto-occipital extension. If cervical spine precautions are not required, assess the patient's ability to flex the neck at the lower part of the cervical spine and extend the head on the upper cervical spine. (PSA should not be performed on a patient with a potential cervical spinal injury except under exigent circumstances.)

Pathology of the upper airway. Assess for evidence of upper airway obstruction resulting from medical causes (e.g. angioedema, tumours, epiglottitis) or traumatic causes (e.g. burns, penetrating neck trauma). The presence of stridor might identify such pathologies.

AMPLE history

The AMPLE mnemonic is useful in your initial patient assessment.

Allergies. It is important to enquire about allergies to medication and/or previous adverse events when the patient has been sedated or undergone anaesthesia.

Medication. Medication that is currently being used must be established. Both allopathic and homeopathic medications may cause drug interactions. The use of chronic medication can reveal a diagnosis that may not have been mentioned previously. Also check whether the patient has taken/been given analgesia/other medication for the current problem prior to hospital arrival.

Past medical history. This would have hopefully been covered in the initial patient evaluation but serves as a reminder.

Last meal. The time since the patient last imbibed solids and liquids may impact on the timing of the procedural sedation (see the section on Fasting, p. 206).

Events/Environment. Having knowledge of the events leading up to the presentation in the ED (e.g. seizure leading to a shoulder dislocation) may influence the choice of drugs and procedure.

Back-up/background

PSA should not be taken lightly. As with all patient interventions, there are benefits as well as potential adverse events of which the physician should be aware. The safety and efficacy of PSA is unequivocal as long as safe practice guidelines are followed. Background knowledge of PSA is fundamental to its sound performance.

Although the goal of procedural sedation is to induce mild to moderate or dissociative sedation, the patient's level of sedation may fluctuate due to individual variations in their response to the medication, so the physician must be competent in the skills required to rescue a patient whose level of sedation becomes deeper than that desired. The physician should also be well versed in the different drug options, their indications and contraindications, and be able to make an appropriate choice for the selected procedure.

Should there be any doubt in the practitioner's mind as to the patient's safety prior to or while performing PSA, its practice should be deferred and an alternative means sought (e.g. procedure performed in the operating theatre).

Back-up equipment, resuscitation equipment and drugs, as well as trained staff should always be at hand in case of an adverse event.

Consent

Informed consent should be obtained from the patient, parent or legal guardian. Ideally, this should be written consent but will depend on the policy of the hospital or department in which you are working.

The patient/parent should be told about the proposed order of events (including the need for post-procedural monitoring prior to discharge), potential complications, and alternative options available to them. Parents must specifically be warned about the changes they may see in their child during the procedural sedation. This is especially true for the effects of dissociative agents such as ketamine, which can commonly cause nystagmus, excessive salivation, non-specific crying (on induction, intra-procedure and on arousal) and strange movements which may be disconcerting for the parents.

Drugs

Knowledge of the pharmacokinetics and pharmacodynamics of the drugs used is paramount to the success of the procedural sedation. There is a variety of drugs that can be used alone or in combination, administered via a range of different routes, in order to achieve the goal of safe and effective procedural sedation.

The ideal drug or drug combination should have a rapid onset of action, a short duration of action, be easily titrated to the desired effect, have a low adverse-effect profile, and be inexpensive. Although this has not been completely attainable to date, certain drugs/combinations have come close.

Children must always be weighed in order to accurately calculate dosages of drugs.

Routes of administration

The route chosen for drug administration will depend on drug availability, patient choice, paediatric considerations, physician choice and familiarity, duration of the procedure, and the volume of drug to be administered.

Drug availability

The ED where you work may not stock a drug that has the option of multiple different routes (e.g. ketamine), or may only have a drug which has to be given intravenously (e.g. propofol).

Patient choice

Children (and some adults) might not consent to the use of a needle for drug administration. The oral or nasal routes might then have to be considered.

Paediatric considerations

A once-off intramuscular injection may be preferred to the 'torture' which may be associated with obtaining intravenous access or the delay in waiting for topical anaesthesia to take effect at a prospective venous access site.

Physician choice and familiarity

This applies to the choice of drug as well as to the route of administration. Despite the security of being accustomed to a certain drug, the best and most appropriate drug for the procedure should be used. The physician practising PSA should become well acquainted at least with etomidate, fentanyl, ketamine, midazolam and propofol.

Duration of procedure

Intravenous administration generally has the quickest onset and duration of action amongst all the possible routes of administration. This is useful for quick procedures and can also be useful to titrate a drug if the procedure becomes prolonged. Intramuscular administration is not as easily titrated or predictable and has a longer duration of onset and time to recovery.

Volume of drug to be administered

Certain medications allow for intranasal or rectal administration. Intranasal administration is usually limited by volume (depending on the formulation of the medication) as well as availability of administration devices.

Sedative agents

Midazolam

Midazolam is the benzodiazepine 'work-horse' of the ED. The beneficial effects of midazolam include good amnesia and anxiolysis, a relatively short onset of action, and multiple possible routes of administration. It also has anticonvulsant and muscle relaxant properties. The duration of action is approximately 30 minutes when given intravenously, which is much longer than the other sedative agents (Table 11.2). Midazolam has no analgesic properties, so should be administered with an opiate for painful procedures. This can prolong the predicted recovery time and increase the potential complications. It can cause respiratory depression but usually does not result in

Table 11.2 Action of midazolam

Route		Dose	Onset	Duration of action
IV	Adult	0.02–0.1 mg/kg	1–2 min	30 min
	Child	0.05–0.15 mg/kg		
IM		0.05–0.15 mg/kg	15–30 min	60–120 min
PO		0.5–0.75 mg/kg	10–30 min	60–90 min
PR		0.5–0.75 mg/kg	10–15 min	45–60 min
Intranasal		0.75–1.0 mg/kg	<1 min	5–10 min

cardiovascular compromise in the comparatively low doses used for PSA. The dose should be halved in elderly patients. Owing to the different pharmacokinetics of midazolam in children, the recommended dose used is slightly higher, but paradoxical agitation is not uncommon.

Propofol

Propofol is an ultra-rapid-acting sedative–hypnotic. It has a very rapid onset, with a duration of action usually less than 10 minutes (Table 11.3). Besides these obvious favourable benefits, propofol is also advantageous because of its antiemetic and anticonvulsant properties. Respiratory depression and apnoea may occur, but are of brief duration and easily remedied by oxygen administration or bag–mask ventilation if necessary. Hypotension is also a frequent occurrence and the drug should therefore be avoided in hypotensive patients. Propofol has no analgesic properties, so should typically be administered with a short-acting opioid. Pain on injection is improved by mixing the drug with a small amount (0.25 mg/kg) of intravenous lidocaine. Propofol is contraindicated in patients who are allergic to egg or soya. Repeated

Table 11.3 Action of propofol

Route	Dose	Onset	Duration of action
IV	1 mg/kg	<1 min	8–10 min

doses may be given at 5-minute intervals as required, at half the initial dose (i.e. 0.5 mg/kg).

Etomidate

Etomidate is a rapidly acting sedative commonly used for rapid sequence intubation in the haemodynamically unstable patient. It approaches the ideal procedural sedation agent because it has a rapid onset of action, short duration of action and a mild adverse effect profile (Table 11.4). It does not have any analgesic properties. Etomidate causes a transient reduction in cerebral blood flow, which is thought to be cerebrally protective. It also has relatively little effect on the cardiovascular system. These features make it a good choice for patients who may be haemodynamically compromised or have raised intracranial pressure. Myoclonus is a common side effect, which can sometimes be mistaken for a seizure. Vomiting and respiratory depression are not uncommon. Etomidate does cause adrenal suppression – controversy exists as to whether this is clinically relevant to the patient's outcome.

Table 11.4 Action of etomidate

Route	Dose	Onset	Duration of action
IV	0.1–0.2 mg/kg	<1 min	5–8 min

Analgesic agents
Fentanyl

Fentanyl is a rapidly acting, high-potency opioid with a short duration of action and favourable side-effect profile (Table 11.5). These features

Table 11.5 Action of fentanyl

Route	Dose	Onset	Duration of action
IV	1 µg/kg	1–2 min	20–30 min
Transmucosal	10–15 µg/kg	15–30 min	60–120 min
Intranasal	1–2 µg/kg	5 min	30–60 min

make it the opioid of choice for PSA. Its versatility is further enhanced by a choice of administration routes – intravenous, oral transmucosal and nasal. Adverse effects include respiratory depression, muscular and glottic rigidity, facial pruritus, nausea and vomiting. Rigidity can be overcome with naloxone or succinylcholine.

Alfentanil

Reports of PSA using this drug have been favourable – it is a high-potency opiate with a shorter half-life than fentanyl. This makes it an extremely good choice for short procedures.

Dissociative agents
Ketamine

The trance-like state induced by ketamine, together with its powerful analgesic properties, make it a unique PSA drug. It has the additional benefits of not causing respiratory depression or muscle relaxation; therefore, patients can still maintain their protective airway reflexes. Although most commonly employed in paediatric procedural sedation, ketamine has been shown to be equally safe in adult patients. Ketamine also has the convenience of multi-route administration (Table 11.6). Ketamine may stimulate salivary and airway secretions (especially in children), but the use of atropine (0.01 mg/kg, minimum dose 0.1 mg, maximum dose 0.5 mg) is not routinely needed. Vomiting and emergence phenomena are common side effects. Aspiration following ketamine is extremely rare though. The agitation that occurs on emergence is generally mild and rarely requires treatment besides reassurance. It

Table 11.6 Action of ketamine

Route	Dose	Onset	Duration of action
IV	1–2 mg/kg	1 min	15 min
IM	3–4 mg/kg	5 min	15–30 min
PO	5–8 mg/kg	30–45 min	2–4 h
PR	5–10 mg/kg	5–10 min	15–30 min
Intranasal	6–10 mg/kg*	5–10 min	15–30 min

*The dose for intranasal use has not been well established.

is so safe, that there are case reports of 10-fold and even 100-fold over-doses in children that have resulted in no major morbidities or mortalities. It should be used with caution in infants younger than 3 months, in patients with pulmonary infections and in patients with cardiovascular disease (angina, cardiac failure, uncontrolled hypertension).

Non-invasive methods

Nitrous oxide

Nitrous oxide (N_2O) is a colourless, sweet-smelling gas and the oldest known anaesthetic agent. It is more commonly used by dentists and as an adjunct in anaesthesia. Nitrous oxide produces sedation, anxiolysis and analgesia in as little as 1 to 2 minutes. Its duration of action is also short – usually 3 to 5 minutes (Table 11.7). The analgesic properties of nitrous oxide are not as potent as its ability to provide sedation and anxiolysis, so for more painful procedures, opioid or local anaesthesia should be administered concurrently. Nitrous oxide is usually administered in concentrations of 30% to 50% in the ED. Owing to changes in partial pressure of the gas, higher concentrations (65% to 70%) are required at high altitude. Hypoxia is avoided by ensuring a minimum of 30% oxygen and close monitoring of the patient's respiratory status. Administering nitrous oxide with an appropriate pre-emptive psychological input has been known to enhance its action and make it more effective at lower doses – for example, if a patient expects to fall asleep whilst inhaling nitrous oxide, they most probably will. Nitrous oxide should be administered in a well-ventilated area, preferably with a scavenger system in place, in order to prevent inhalation by ED staff. It is a known teratogen, so care should be exercised around pregnant patients and staff members. The best way of using nitrous oxide is via a self-administered mask with a demand-valve. This means that the patient needs to hold the mask to their face and generate 3 to 5 cm H_2O of negative pressure in order to allow gas to flow. If the patient becomes too sedated, they will not be able to generate the negative pressure, or

Table 11.7 Action of nitrous oxide			
Route	Dose	Onset	Duration of action
Inhalation	30–70%	1–2 min	3–5 min

the mask may fall away, which will stop the delivery of the gas. Unfortunately, this technique does not work well in paediatric patients or those who are not cooperative. Nausea and vomiting are common adverse effects.

Contraindications
- Diseases sensitive to air pressure changes, e.g. intracranial air, bowel obstruction, middle ear disease, decompression sickness, bullous lung diseases, air embolism.
- Decreased level of consciousness.
- Pregnancy.
- Vitamin B_{12} or folate deficiency.
- Immunosuppression.
- Significant cardiac failure.

Sucrose

Mary Poppins was right – a 'spoonful of sugar' does help the 'medicine go down'. This is especially true in infants less than 6 months of age, where 2 mL of a 24% oral sucrose solution (1 teaspoon of sugar in 20 mL of water) reduces the signs of distress caused by minor painful procedures. The usefulness of sucrose diminishes in infants older than 6 months. The efficacy of sucrose is enhanced in combination with non-nutritive sucking such as sucking on a pacifier. The sucrose is most effective when given approximately 2 minutes before the invasive procedure is attempted.

Equipment and monitoring

Appropriately trained personnel, correct equipment and adequate monitoring are integral for the safe administration of PSA.

Appropriately trained personnel

The minimum required personnel to safely administer PSA are a doctor and a registered nurse. It is safe for the same doctor to perform the PSA and the procedure. Should the procedure to be performed be complex and require the doctor's full attention throughout, a second doctor should be brought in to monitor the patient's clinical status during the procedure. The nurse must remain monitoring the patient after the procedure until the patient is fully awake and ready for discharge.

The doctor performing the procedural sedation must be competent in the skills required to rescue a patient from a level of sedation deeper than the desired level.

Equipment

All equipment that may be required for the PSA process as well as all resuscitation equipment must be checked and available at the patient's bedside should there be any sedation-related complications. This includes:

- Equipment for supporting the airway and ventilation (oxygen masks/nasal cannulae, appropriately sized bag–mask, laryngoscope, endotracheal tubes, bougie, suction and rescue devices, e.g. laryngeal mask airway).
- Drugs for resuscitation, anaphylaxis and antidotes/reversal agents.
- A defibrillator.

Oxygen

The routine use of supplemental oxygen in PSA is debatable. On the one hand it is thought that it might cause a delay in detecting hypoventilation, as the patient's oxygen saturation is maintained longer by the supplemental oxygen administration. On the other hand, drug-induced apnoea in a well-oxygenated patient is less likely to be troublesome.

Monitoring

Constant clinical assessment and vital signs monitoring are core principles in procedural sedation. Vital signs should be monitored continually. Documentation of the patient's level of consciousness, heart rate, blood pressure, respiratory rate and oxygen saturation should be recorded pre-procedure and then every 5 minutes until the patient has recovered.

Pulse oximetry

Pulse oximetry is a valuable method of monitoring the patient continuously and non-invasively. It is reliable in detecting decreases in oxygen saturation as well as changes in the patient's heart rate. The limitation of pulse oximetry is in detecting early decreases in ventilation. A patient may develop hypoventilation, but a drop in the oxygen saturation will lag behind the onset of hypercarbia and apnoea. The concomitant administration of oxygen is also thought to mask this hypoventilation by delaying the detection of decreased oxygen saturation. Therefore, continuous clinical monitoring must be used in conjunction with pulse oximetry.

Capnometry

Hypoventilation is a common side effect of both the sedative and analgesic drugs used in procedural sedation. This can be identified earlier by non-invasively monitoring the patient's end-tidal carbon dioxide ($ETCO_2$) level. An increase in $ETCO_2$ will detect inadequate ventilation earlier than oxygen desaturation would. The normal range for $ETCO_2$ is between 40 and 48 mmHg.

Fasting

Conventional pre-operative guidelines promulgated by the ASA for patients undergoing general anaesthesia recommend a minimum *nulla per os* (NPO) period of 6 hours for solids, 4 hours for breast milk, and 2 hours for clear liquids. The idea behind this thinking is to prevent aspiration of gastric contents into the lungs, even though there is insufficient data to establish a cause-and-effect relationship between NPO times and adverse outcome prevention. These fasting guidelines have unfortunately been extrapolated to the ED for PSA, despite the very different environment and procedure to be performed. Whereas general anaesthesia routinely involves airway manipulation, which is known to increase the aspiration risk, PSA aims to have the patient maintain their own airway reflexes with no manipulation thereof. Studies have shown that aspiration is not linked to NPO times, so, whereas it is mandatory in general anaesthesia, fasting is a consideration but *not a necessity* for ED PSA.

The timing of the patient's last meal should be documented. The risks of the sedation and remote possibility of aspiration must be balanced against the benefits of performing the procedure promptly and individualised to the patient and the situation.

Guidelines for discharge

The determination of discharge readiness should be individualised for each patient in order to ensure that the patient will not experience any serious or life-threatening adverse event at home.

The decision-making process should include the following criteria:

- Stable vital signs.
- The airway is open and protected.
- Age-appropriate responses back to baseline.
- Adequate hydration.
- Must be supervised and/or able to understand discharge instructions.

The clinician must also take into account the sedative and/or analgesic agent used, the route of administration and the duration of action, as well as whether any adverse events were experienced during the procedure.

The aim is to ensure early safe discharge from the ED; however, if any doubt exists as to the condition of the patient, it is better to err on the side of prolonged observation than premature discharge.

Summary

PSA has been devised based on demand and need. Pressure on theatre lists and the risks of general anaesthesia have created a niche for the practice of safe and effective PSA in the ED. A structured approach, adequate training and meticulous pre-procedural preparation will ensure the safety and satisfaction of both patient and doctor alike.

In summary, these elements are applied to the provision of PSA by means of a plan which consists of the following sequential steps:

Step 1   Decide what form of PSA is most appropriate for the procedure to be performed.

Step 2   Perform the baseline focused patient assessment, confirm that the necessary back-up is available, and re-evaluate the patient's background to ensure that they are eligible for safe PSA.

Step 3   Obtain written informed consent for both the procedure and the PSA.

Step 4   Brief the staff members involved and the patient and/or family on the plan of action and the safety protocols. Check the equipment and connect the monitoring devices. Measure the weight of the patient and calculate the required doses (and dilutions if necessary) of medications.

Step 5   Administer the selected analgesic agent first, followed a short while later by titration of the sedative agent. If an opiate is given after the sedative medication, the incidence of oversedation is higher.

Step 6   Monitor oxygen saturations and heart rate continuously (and end-tidal CO_2 if available). Monitor blood pressure and depth of sedation regularly.

Step 7   Once the procedure is completed, the patient must be monitored until they have fully recovered from the PSA and it is safe to discharge them with written discharge instructions.

Case studies

The ABCDEFG methodology applies to all patients who are to undergo PSA. Each case needs to be considered individually as to whether sedation, analgesia, regional anaesthesia or a combination thereof needs to be employed in order to facilitate the performance of a potentially unpleasant procedure. There will be variability amongst different healthcare practitioners as to their approach used for different procedures. No one option is necessarily better than another, as long as patient safety and comfort is the ultimate aim. The examples below are potential approaches which may be used for these typical scenarios.

Case 1

A 36-year-old, 75 kg male has been stabbed in his right chest. He is taken through to the ED. In the resuscitation room, the patient is attached to monitoring equipment, has oxygen administered and peripheral intravenous cannulation performed. The patient is diagnosed with a right-sided haemopneumothorax on x-ray. The consultant Emergency Physician tells the medical officer managing the case that the patient will require an intercostal drain (ICD) to be inserted.

The nurse reports that his vital signs are as follows:

Blood pressure	121/68 mmHg
Pulse	82 beats per minute
Respiratory rate	22 breaths per minute
Pulse oximetry	99% on a partial rebreather mask at 15 L/min

The patient is assessed by the medical officer to be ASA class 2 with a Mallampati class I airway and no signs of being potentially difficult to bag–mask ventilate or intubate. He has no allergies or previous medical or surgical history. His last meal was 4 hours ago. Verbal consent is obtained for PSA as well as for the insertion of the ICD.

The patient is given 75 µg of fentanyl intravenously and a 500 mL fluid bolus. The medical officer performs an intercostal block with 1% lidocaine. Three minutes later, 75 mg of propofol is slowly titrated intravenously over 1 minute. The intercostal drain is inserted uneventfully and 400 mL of blood drains into the bottle. The patient is monitored for 30 minutes post-procedure. He required a further 500 mL crystalloid fluid bolus but remained haemodynamically stable. He was awake and oriented, and given an intrapleural block with 0.5% bupivacaine before being transferred to the ward.

Case 2

A 6-year-old, 20 kg girl falls off the jungle-gym whilst playing at school. She comes into the ED crying, complaining of pain in her left wrist. An x-ray reveals a markedly angulated greenstick fracture of her left distal radius and ulna. The registrar on duty elects to use PSA in order to facilitate manipulation and splinting of the fracture. The patient is known to be a well-controlled asthmatic and is currently in good health. She last ate a meal 3 hours ago. Evaluation of her airway yields no disconcerting features. The patient is categorised as ASA class 2. The procedure is explained to the parents and written consent is obtained. EMLA cream had already been applied to the right antecubital fossa 1 hour previously, when the patient was initially triaged. An intravenous cannula is painlessly inserted and the young girl is taken through to the procedure room and attached to monitoring equipment. The registrar had checked the presence of resuscitation equipment and drug availability when she came on duty that morning. The child is given 20 mg of ketamine slowly intravenously. After 1 minute, she has nystagmus and is breathing spontaneously with adequate vital signs. The fracture is manipulated and a splint applied. The child cries briefly during the manipulation only. After 45 minutes, the patient is sleepy but arousable enough to be sent for a control x-ray accompanied by her parents. On her return, she is awake and communicative. The parents are given a copy of the discharge instructions and told to return should there be any concerns. Four weeks later, the child returns for a check-up. She runs towards the doctor and hugs her – thanking her for fixing her arm.

Case 3

A 62-year-old, 50 kg female slips on wet tiles at the supermarket and presents to the ED with an isolated anterior dislocation of her left shoulder. The patient is on various medications for her rheumatoid arthritis and hypertension. She is allergic to soya. The patient is assessed to be ASA class 3. She is a Mallampati class II but has severe limitation of movement of her atlanto-occipital joint due to the rheumatoid arthritis. In view of the patient's chronic illness and frailty, the doctor opts to reduce the shoulder with a short-acting opioid and local anaesthesia.

He injects 20 mL of 0.5% lidocaine into the subacromial space under sterile conditions. After 20 minutes, he gives 25 μg of fentanyl. After waiting a further 2 minutes, he attempts to reduce the shoulder by scapular manipulation. He succeeds after the second attempt. The patient is monitored until fully conscious and discharged back to the retirement village in the care of her daughter.

Case 4

A 45-year-old, 80 kg male patient requires a computed tomography (CT) scan of his brain because of a seizure following a head injury. He is claustrophobic and terrified of entering the CT scanner. He has no alarming features on the focused assessment.

The Emergency Physician administers a small dose (2 mg) of lorazepam intravenously to induce minimal sedation (anxiolysis), after which the patient calmly submits to the CT examination. He requires no supplemental oxygen and the saturations remain above 95%. One hour after the CT scan, he can safely be discharged home in the company of his wife as he is fully awake and alert with an intact airway.

RECOMMENDED READING

Useful websites

The NYSORA – New York School of Regional Anesthesia website is an excellent resource for information on conventional nerve-stimulator and ultrasound-guided techniques. It also has an excellent section on oral and dental local anaesthesia. The images and quality of information are superb. http://nysora.com/

The 'Family practice notebook' has useful titbits of information. There are some helpful, simple bits of information on selected blind nerve blocks in the site. It is worth a visit for the novice nerve-blocker. http://www.fpnotebook.com/Surgery/Pharm/index.htm

The AnaesthesiaUK website has an enormous amount of information on all aspects of anaesthesia, including regional anaesthesia. There is comprehensive information on the anatomy, preparation and performance of nerve blocks using the nerve stimulator as well as ultrasound. The link provided is to the section on regional anaesthesia. http://www.frca.co.uk/SectionContents.aspx?sectionid=173

'Ultrasound for regional anesthesia' has a wealth of information on the general application of ultrasound in regional anaesthesia as well as specific nerve-block techniques. It will provide all the information needed to confidently attempt any of the procedures. http://www.usra.ca/

The Sonosite website is a commercial website that sells instructional video clips on ultrasound-guided regional nerve blockade. These clips can be downloaded from this site (at a cost). http://sonositelearning.com/clinical_applications/anesthesiology/

'Peripheral regional anaesthesia', edited by Professor HH Mehrkens of the Anaesthesiology Department of the Ulm Rehabilitation Hospital, provides a slightly different approach to various common nerve blocks and makes for interesting reading. This website describes nerve-stimulator techniques only. http://www.nerveblocks.net/

'Neuraxiom.com ultrasound guided nerve blocks' is a wonderful site created by Jack vander Beek. This author is a straight-speaking proponent of ultrasound-guided nerve blocks. He is also clearly an expert and deep thinker on this subject and his website is a must-visit for both the novice and expert. There is a wealth of information on this site. http://www.neuraxiom.com/

The Dartmouth-Hitchcock Medical Center's Center for Ultrasound-Guided Regional Anesthesia website has a to-the-point brief description of each important block. The video clips and images are useful for self-education. http://www.dhmc.org/webpage.cfm?site_id=2&org_id=594&gsec_id=0&sec_id=0&item_id=33614

The Chinese University of Hong Kong's website for ultrasound-guided regional anaesthesia has a large amount of information on nerve blocks. The videos and images are a useful adjunct to the teaching material. http://www.usgraweb.hk

Selected references

Barnett P: Alternatives to sedation for painful procedures, *Pediatr Emerg Care* 25(6):415–419; quiz 420–422, 2009.

Becker DE, Reed KL: Essentials of local anesthetic pharmacology, *Anesth Prog* 53(3):98–108, 2006.

Blaivas M, Lyon M: Ultrasound-guided interscalene block for shoulder dislocation reduction in the ED, *Am J Emerg Med* 24(3):293–296, 2006.

Chong AK, Tan DM, Ooi BS, Mahadevan M, Lim AY, Lim BH: Comparison of forearm and conventional Bier's blocks for manipulation and reduction of distal radius fractures, *J Hand Surg Eur Vol* 32(1):57–59, 2007.

Constantine E, Steele DW, Eberson C, Boutis K, Amanullah S, Linakis JG: The use of local anesthetic techniques for closed forearm fracture reduction in children: a survey of academic pediatric emergency departments, *Pediatr Emerg Care* 23(4):209–211, 2007.

Crystal CS, Blankenship RB: Local anesthetics and peripheral nerve blocks in the emergency department, *Emerg Med Clin North Am* 23(2):477–502, 2005.

Crystal CS, McArthur TJ, Harrison B: Anesthetic and procedural sedation techniques for wound management, *Emerg Med Clin North Am* 25(1): 41–71, 2007.

Crystal CS, Miller MA, Young SE: Ultrasound guided hematoma block: a novel use of ultrasound in the traumatized patient, *J Trauma* 62(2):532–533, 2007.

De Tran QH, Clemente A, Doan J, Finlayson RG: Brachial plexus blocks: a review of approaches and techniques, *Can J Anaesth* 54(8):662–674, 2007.

De Tran QH, Russo G, Muñoz L, Zaouter C, Finlayson RJ: A prospective, randomized comparison between ultrasound-guided supraclavicular, infraclavicular, and axillary brachial plexus blocks, *Reg Anesth Pain Med* 34(4):366–371, 2009.

Dillon D, Gibbs MA, Baby C: Peripheral nerve blocks of the hand, *Acad Emerg Med* 14(1):14–15, 2007.

Ecoffey C: Pediatric regional anesthesia – update, *Curr Opin Anaesthesiol* 20(3):232–235, 2007.

Ferrera PC, Chandler R: Anesthesia in the emergency setting: Part II. Head and neck, eye and rib injuries, *Am Fam Physician* 50(4):797–800, 1994.

Fredrickson MJ: Ultrasound-guided ankle block, *Anaesth Intensive Care* 37(1):143–144, 2009.

Harness NG: Digital block anesthesia, *J Hand Surg Am* 34(1):142–145, 2009.

Jackson LM, Hill RJ: Hill block, a modification of the Bier block, *J Clin Anesth* 18(5):397–398, 2006.

Klaastad O, Sauter AR, Dodgson MS: Brachial plexus block with or without ultrasound guidance, *Curr Opin Anaesthesiol* 22(5):655–660, 2009.

Krombach J, Gray AT: Sonography for saphenous nerve block near the adductor canal, *Reg Anesth Pain Med* 32(4):369–370, 2007. Erratum in: *Reg Anesth Pain Med* 32(6):536, 2007.

Liebmann O, Price D, Mills C, et al: Feasibility of forearm ultrasonography-guided nerve blocks of the radial, ulnar, and median nerves for hand procedures in the emergency department, *Ann Emerg Med* 48(5):558–562, 2006.

Loryman B, Davies F, Chavada G, Coats T: Consigning "brutacaine" to history: a survey of pharmacological techniques to facilitate painful procedures in children in emergency departments in the UK, *Emerg Med J* 23(11):838–840, 2006.

May G, Bartram T: Towards evidence based emergency medicine: best BETs from the Manchester Royal Infirmary. The use of intrapleural anaesthetic to reduce the pain of chest drain insertion, *Emerg Med J* 24(4):300–301, 2007.

Mutty CE, Jensen EJ, Manka MA Jr, Anders MJ, Bone LB: Femoral nerve block for diaphyseal and distal femoral fractures in the emergency department. Surgical technique, *J Bone Joint Surg Am* 90(Suppl 2 Pt 2):218–226, 2008.

O'Sullivan R, Oakley E, Starr M: Wound repair in children, *Aust Fam Physician* 35(7):476–479, 2006.

Ota J, Sakura S, Hara K, Saito Y: Ultrasound-guided anterior approach to sciatic nerve block: a comparison with the posterior approach, *Anesth Analg* 108(2):660–665, 2009.

Perlas A, Brull R, Chan VW, McCartney CJ, Nuica A, Abbas S: Ultrasound guidance improves the success of sciatic nerve block at the popliteal fossa, *Reg Anesth Pain Med* 33(3):259–265, 2008.

Powell SL, Robertson L, Doty BJ: Dental nerve blocks: toothache remedies for the acute-care setting, *Postgrad Med* 107(1):229–245, 2000.

Quaba O, Huntley JS, Bahia H, McKeown DW: A users guide for reducing the pain of local anaesthetic administration, *Emerg Med J* 22(3):188–189, 2005.

Reid N, Stella J, Ryan M, Ragg M: Use of ultrasound to facilitate accurate femoral nerve block in the emergency department, *Emerg Med Australas* 21(2):124–130, 2009.

Salam GA: Regional anesthesia for office procedures: Part I. Head and neck surgeries, *Am Fam Physician* 69(3):585–590, 2004.

Sandeman DJ, Dilley AV: Ultrasound guided dorsal penile nerve block in children, *Anaesth Intensive Care* 35(2):266–269, 2007.

Shen JJ, Taylor DM, Knott JC, MacBean CE: Bupivacaine in the emergency department is underused: scope for improved patient care, *Emerg Med J* 24(3):189–193, 2007.

Socransky SJ, Toner LV: Intra-articular lidocaine for the reduction of posterior shoulder dislocation, *CJEM* 7(6):423–426, 2005.

Stone MB, Price DD, Wang R: Ultrasound-guided supraclavicular block for the treatment of upper extremity fractures, dislocations, and abscesses in the ED, *Am J Emerg Med* 25(4):472–475, 2007.

Tran D, Clemente A, Finlayson RJ: A review of approaches and techniques for lower extremity nerve blocks, *Can J Anaesth* 54(11):922–934, 2007.

INDEX